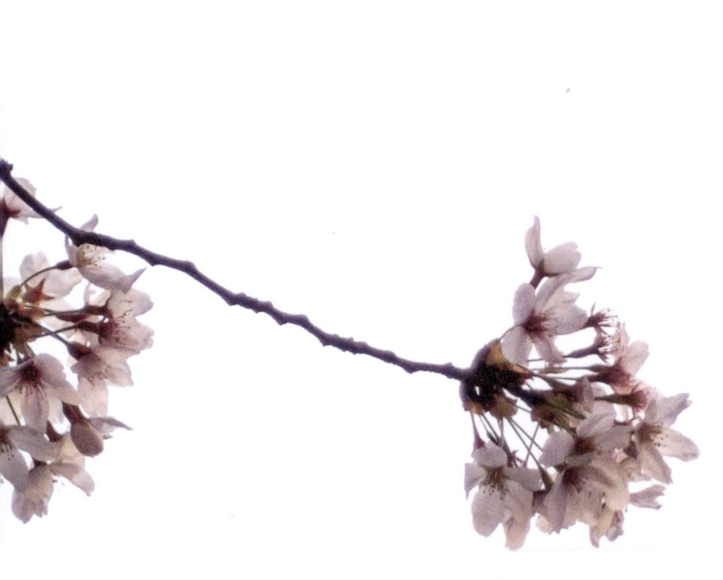

Connection XX

THE FUTURE IS YOURS

THERE IS NO ONE BETTER

Start each day with a grateful heart.

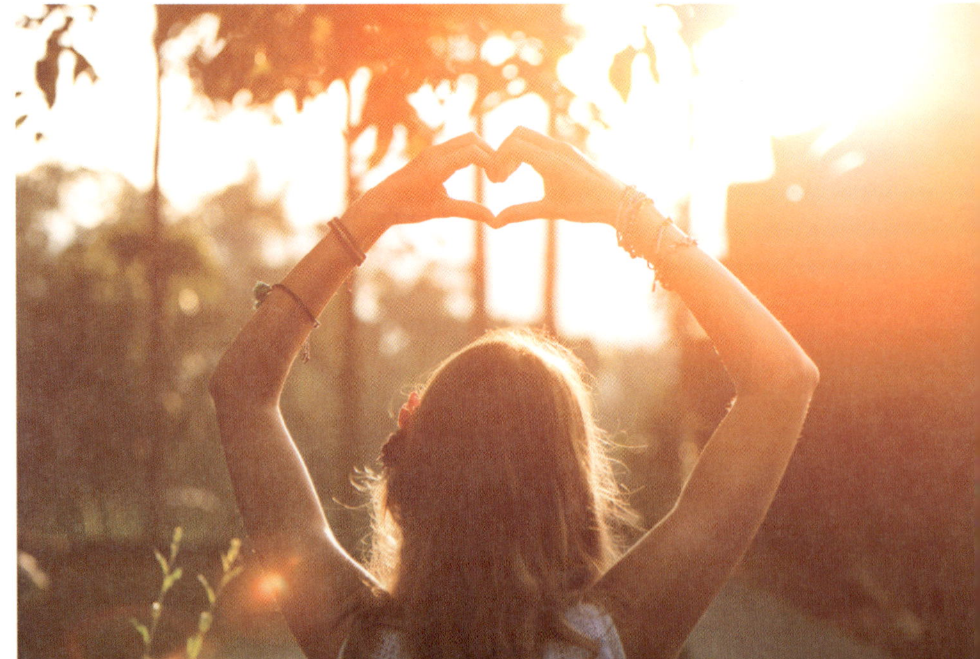

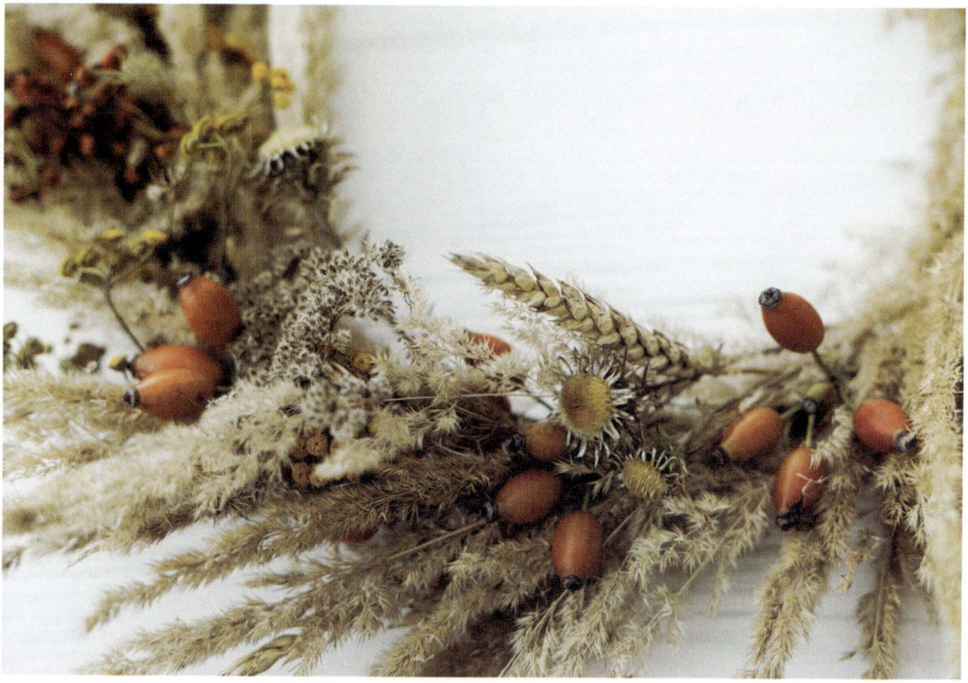

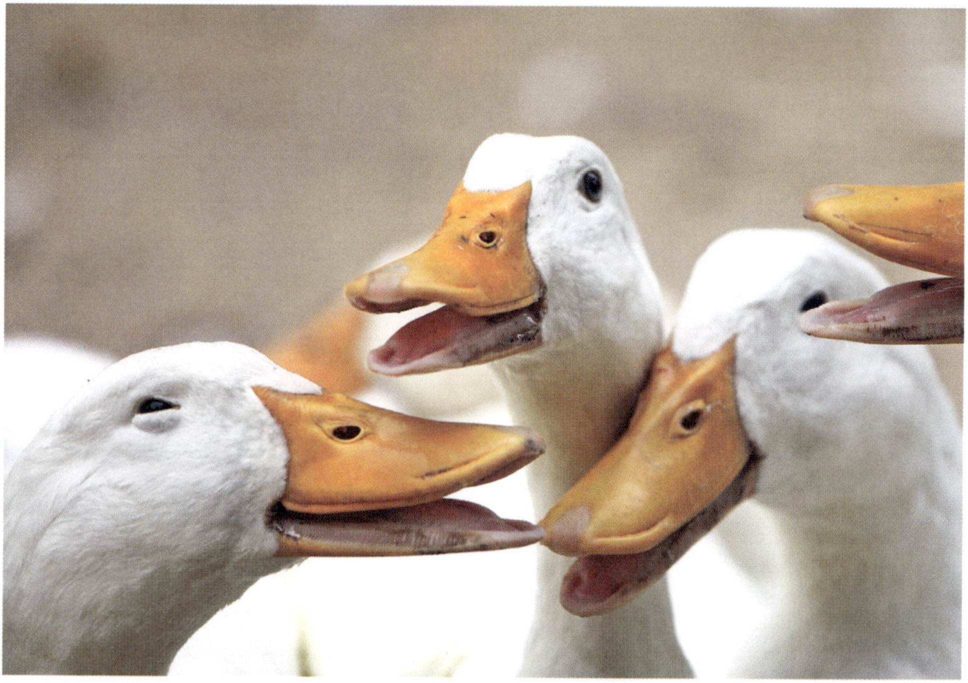

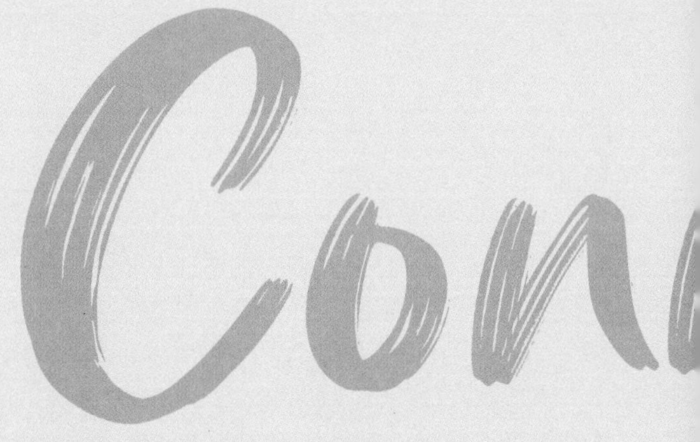

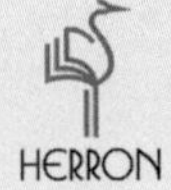
HERRON

DREAM BELIEVER

YOU ARE WHAT YOU IMAGINE

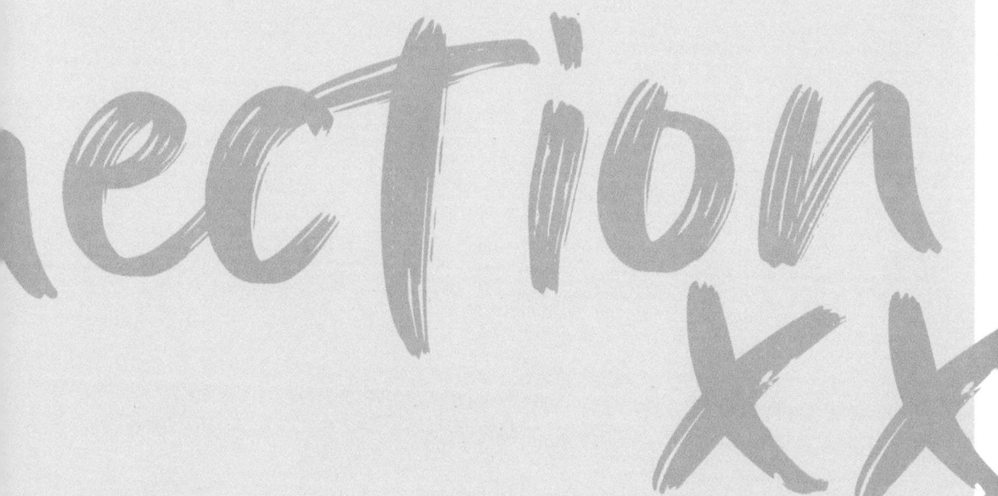

CONTENTS

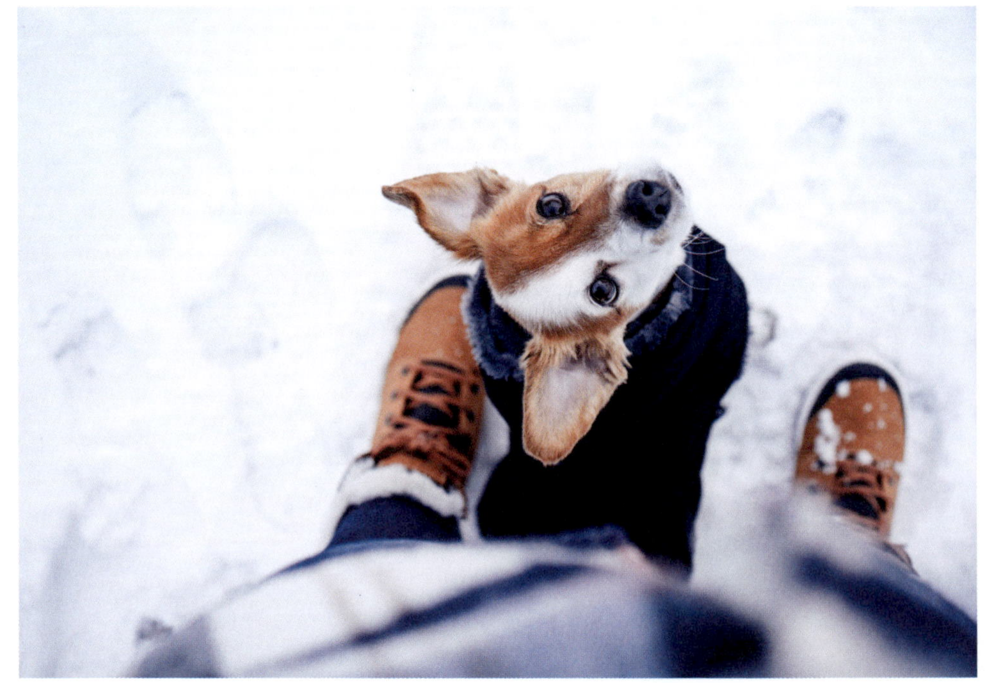

1.

KNOW YOUR TRIBE

2.

PRACTISE EMPATHY

3.

OWN IT

4.

CONNECT DEEPLY

5.

DISCONNECT

Listen with curiosity.

Speak with honesty.

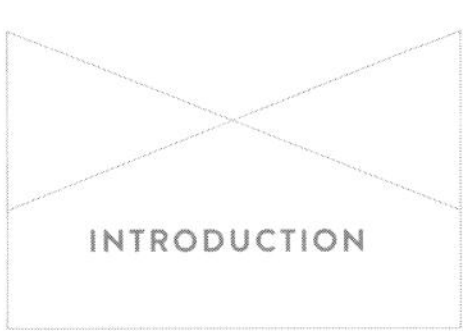

INTRODUCTION

You need connection.

Connecting with others is a basic human need. It's right up there after the basics of food, water, air and safety. We need to feel like we are a part of something, that we belong.

Connection is that moment when an interaction between people leaves each feeling valued, seen and heard. There's no judgement. Each person feels nourished, stronger.

As we grow, we interact and connect with others who help us discover who we are and where we come from. Our family, friends, neighbours, schoolmates and colleagues. Everyone you meet changes you a little and helps you to grow towards who you are going to be. And you help them.

Treasure and nurture the special people in your life. Relationships are like plants – they need attention and care to thrive. Water your relationships with empathy – listen with generosity and imagine yourself in the place of others to feel as they feel.

Making a real connection requires honesty, openness and authenticity. It's not always easy. But like a garden, you'll get out what you put in. Do the hard work, tend to it with care, and it will offer you a lush, peaceful haven, a blissful refuge from the world outside.

To build a beautiful garden, you first need to know the borders of your land. Your boundaries are where you draw the line in relationships, how emotionally close you let people get to you. It's important to have them, and it's just as important to let others know if they are not respecting them.

Your boundaries are ultimately about self-awareness and self-respect – honour them, and you honour yourself.

On the flip side, being open and speaking your truth with other people can be scary. We all carry that fear of rejection, that we'll say or do something stupid and lose face.

Acknowledging that vulnerability and putting ourselves out there anyway is the price of building intimate relationships based on love and respect. It's the everyday bravery of connection.

Finding the balance in relationships between protecting yourself and opening yourself up is not always easy to find. It might take a while to get right. The best thing you can do is explore your feelings and listen to your inner voice – the exercises in this book will help.

"A dream you dream alone is only a dream. A dream you dream together is reality."

– YOKO ONO

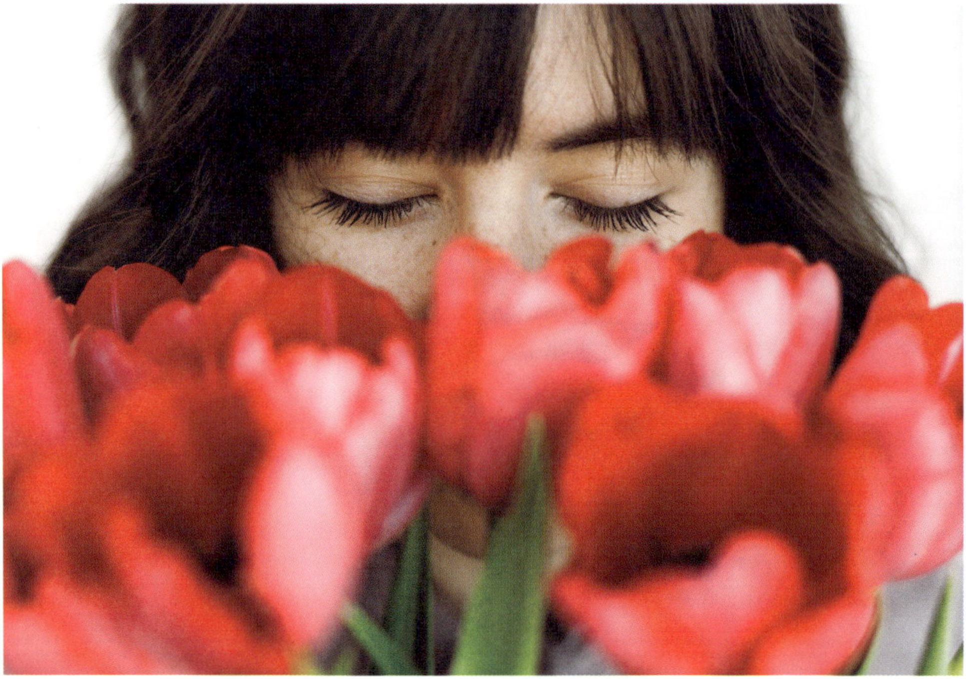

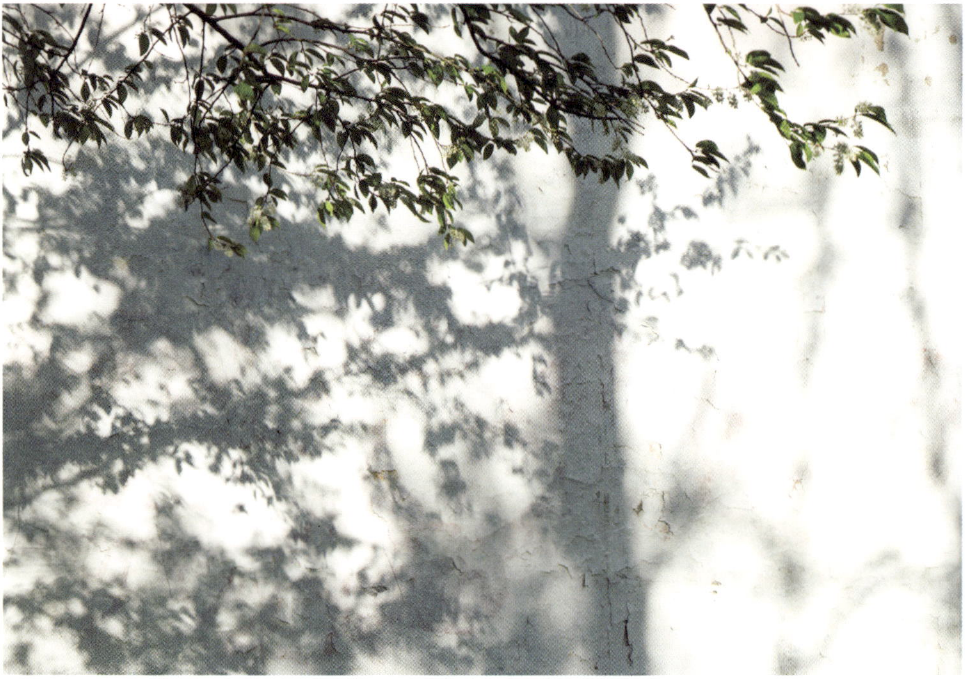

Compassion is the greatest form of love.

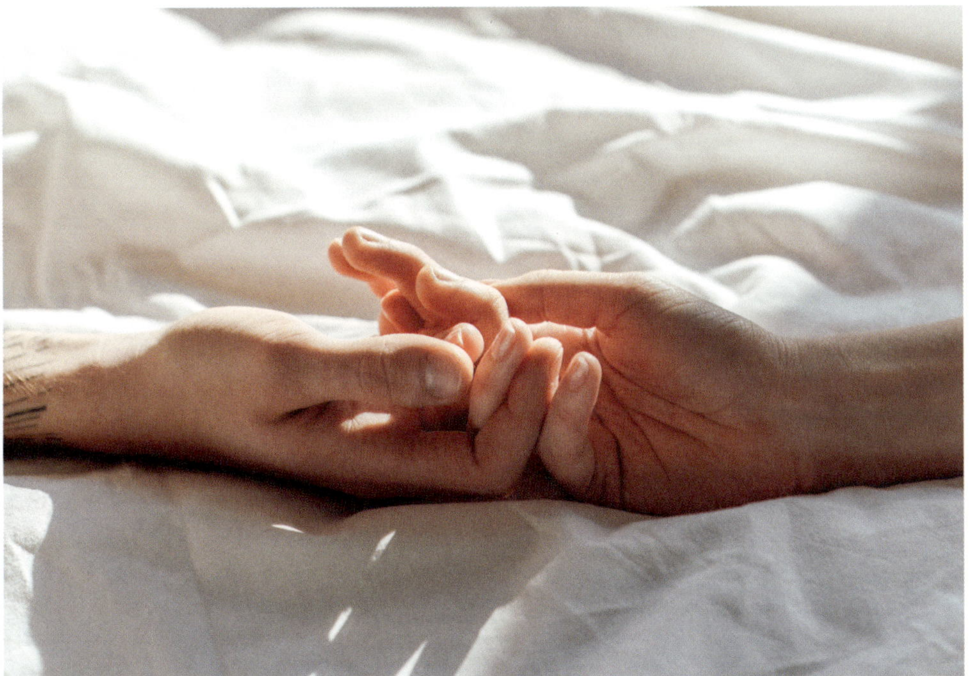

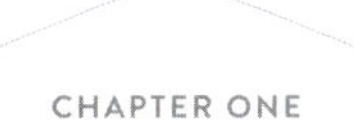

CHAPTER ONE

Know Your Tribe xx

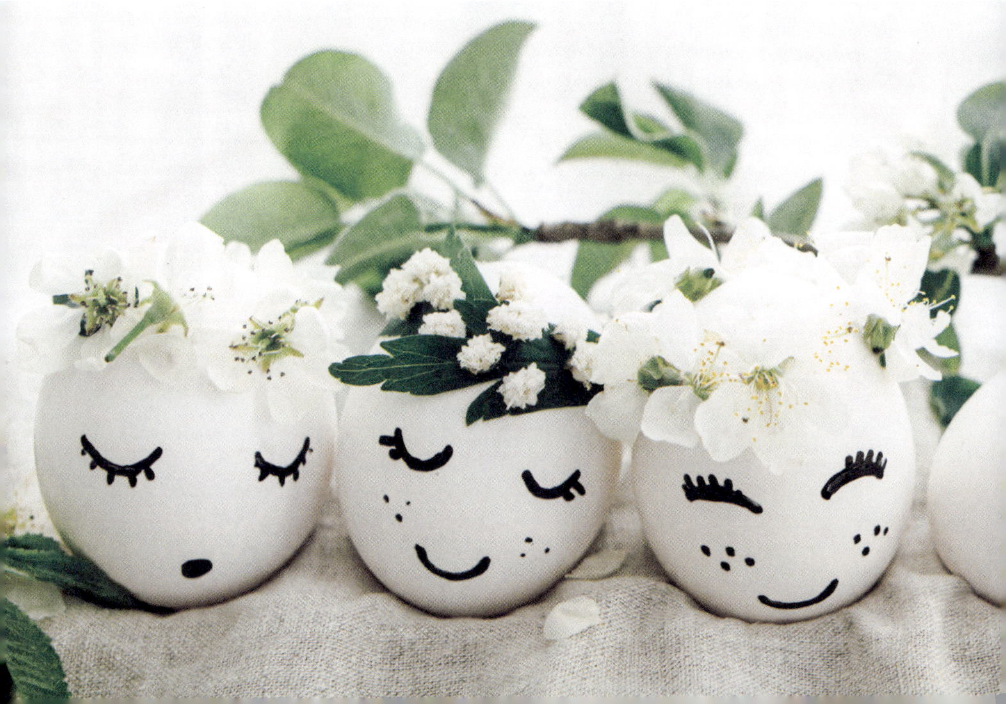

"It is not so much our friends' help that helps us, as the confidence of their help."

EPICURUS

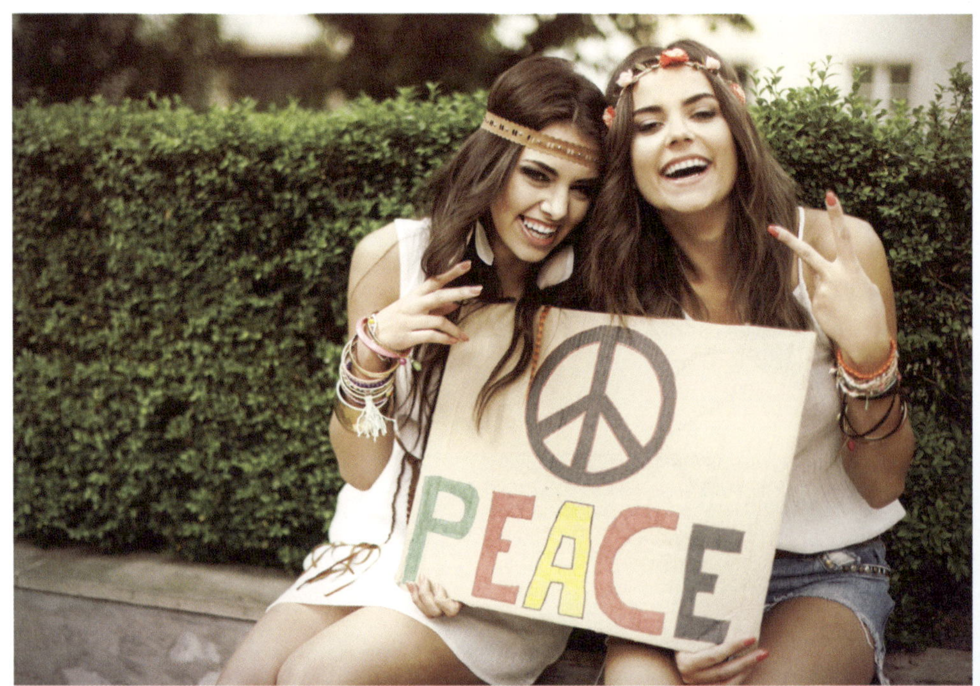

Vibe your tribe

Who's your tribe?

We all need to feel like we're part of something. Having people around us who we identify with, who make us feel we belong, is a basic life necessity.

Think about your tribe. Those closest to you, who you rely on for help and who you're always there for, the ones you call first when something good (or bad) happens, the ones you can be your most authentic self with.

This is probably your closest group of friends. Your family. Now cast the net wider – family friends, teachers, work colleagues, neighbours and others in your community. This is your extended tribe, the many layers of connection you have in your life.

Feeling connected makes us happier, healthier and kinder. Building and nurturing connections, both close and more casual, helps us feel supported, secure and resilient. Other people are our power.

What tribe means to me

Use this section to explore the meaning of tribe. Create your own definition of the concept. What or who is important when you think about the idea of tribe? Write about how it is expressed in your life.

My definition of tribe is …

"Surround yourself only with people who are going to take you higher."

OPRAH WINFREY

It makes me think of (people) ...

I experience it when ...

My tribe map

What does your tribe look like? Make it visual on the page opposite. Place yourself in the centre, with circles of connection starting close to you, like family and friends, and radiating out to more distant (but still important) people in your personal community like neighbours, teachers, sports coaches, family friends and others.

"You become like the five people you spend the most time with. Choose carefully."

JIM ROHN

Changing places

Relationships change. It's normal. As you go through life, relationships will ebb and flow – people will become closer and then further away, new people will enter your tribe, others may gradually move out of it. Think of someone who has been in your life for a long time and write about how your relationship with them has changed. Why do you think these changes have happened? How do you feel about them?

My current relationship with this person is ...

It has changed …

because …

It makes me feel …

Try to put yourself in the other person's place too. How do you think they feel about the changes?

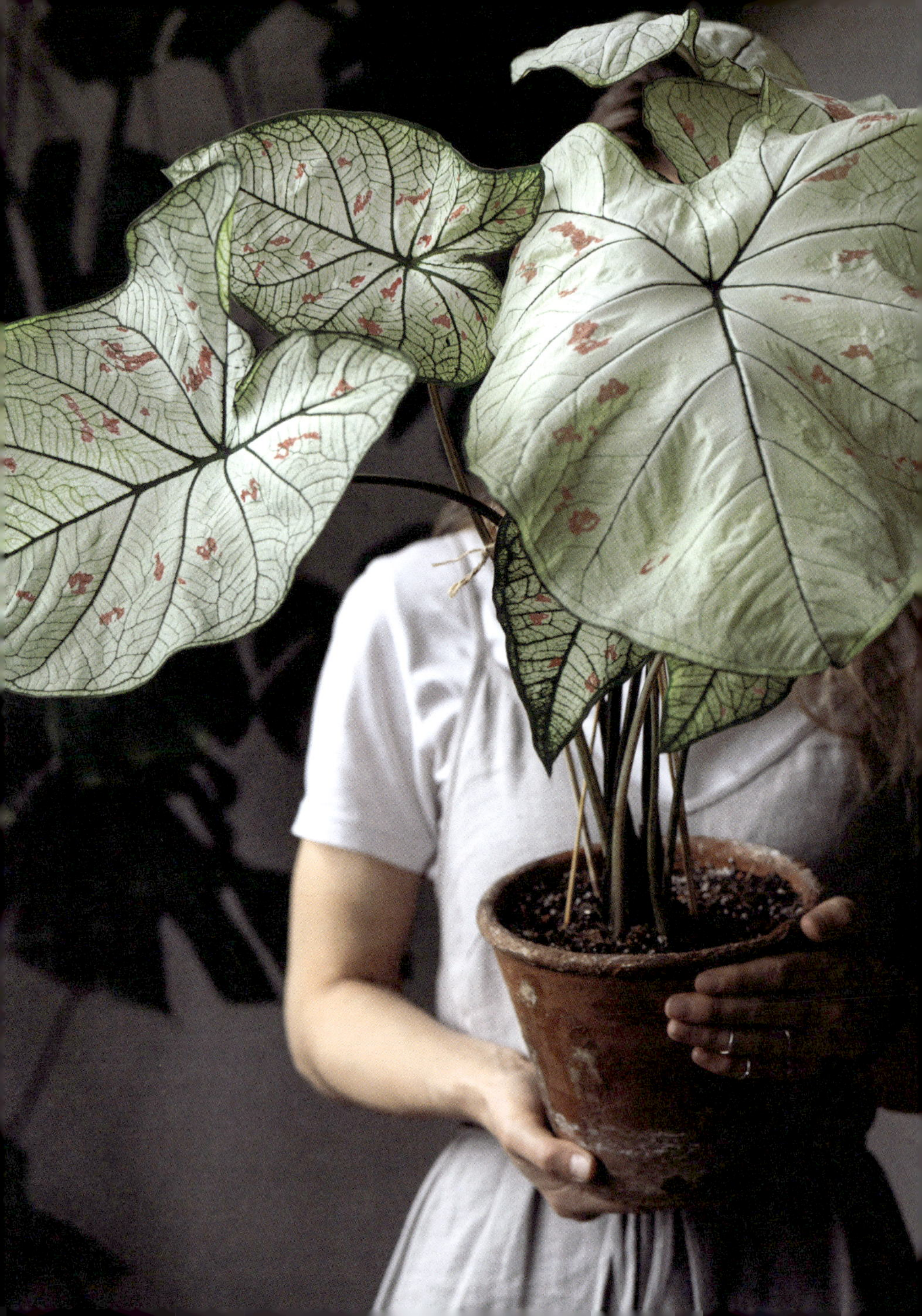

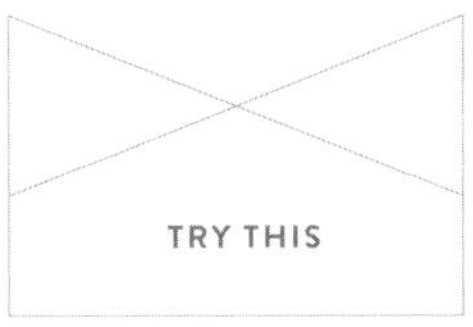

Be a Gardener

Plants need to be nurtured, just like relationships.

Gardening is good for the soul. It can make you feel more peaceful, reduce stress and give your self-esteem a boost when you see the results of your efforts start to bloom.

Looking after your plants, protecting and nurturing them – even talking to them! – supports the qualities of patience and care important for your relationships with others. Cultivate them as you cultivate your little patch of green.

HOW TO DO IT

Start small, with a window box or a few indoor plants. Choose your plants carefully – easy-care varieties are best for beginners. Look online for care instructions, make sure they get enough sun, and don't forget to water!

Thanks, friends

You have a lot to be grateful for when you have a tribe. Support, learning, good times ... Simply the knowledge that there are people to catch you when you fall can boost your confidence and positivity.

Be sure to honour the gifts and growth they bring you. Try to find some time each day to reflect and be grateful for their support.

Even better, write gratitude letters. (Think of it as a thank-you note if that sounds too serious.) When someone does something nice, take the time to let them know how much it meant to you. Be specific about what they did and how it made you feel. It doesn't have to be long – it just has to be heartfelt. If it's on pretty stationery, even better. And if all you can manage is a text message, that's still good!

Even if you don't send the letter, write it anyway. Putting your gratitude in writing will make it more real and more precious.

"Feeling gratitude and not expressing it is like wrapping a present and not giving it."

WILLIAM ARTHUR WARD

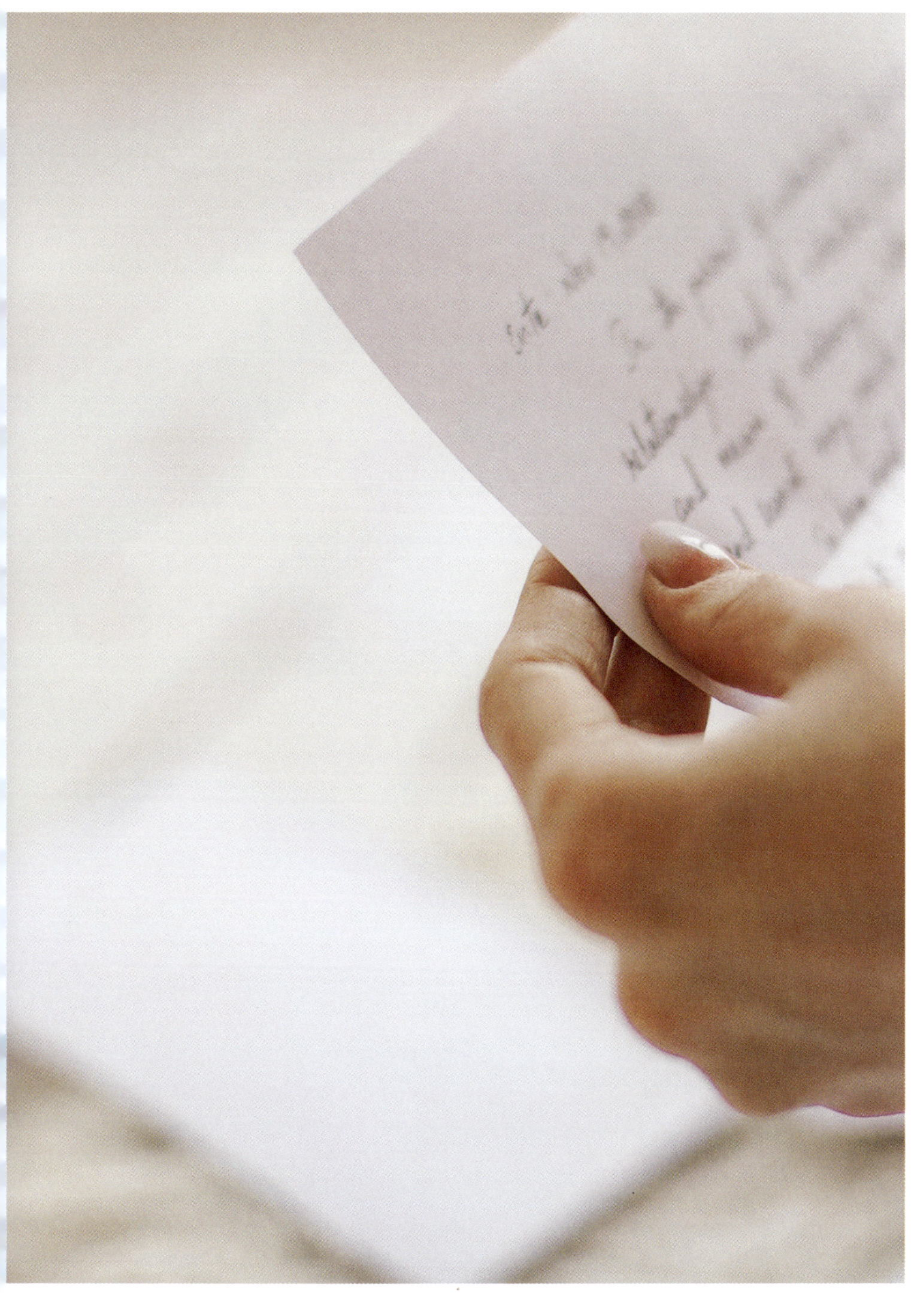

“Show me your friends and I’ll show you your future.”

— MARK AMBROSE

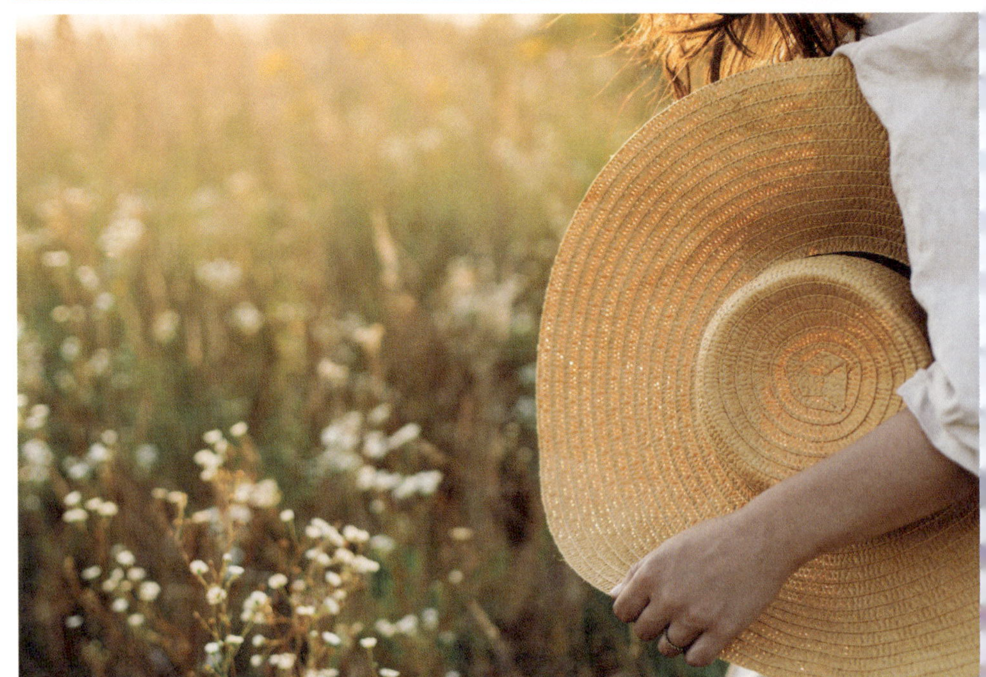

TOOLKIT

Know Your Tribe

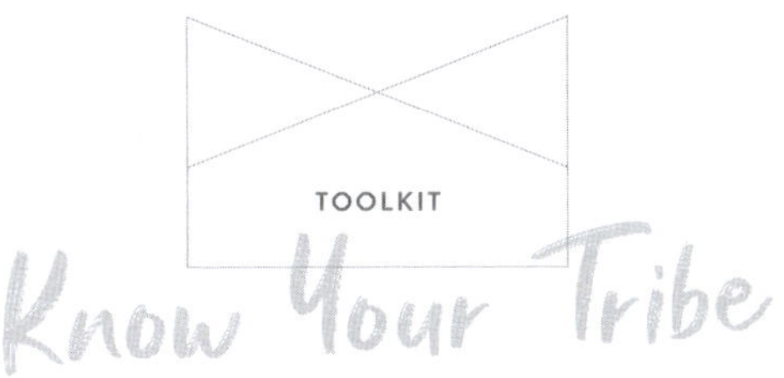

Treasure your tribe with the help of straight-talking turquoise, joyful breaths, caring chamomile and a romantic symbol of enduring love.

AFFIRMATION

I speak my truth with honesty and clarity.

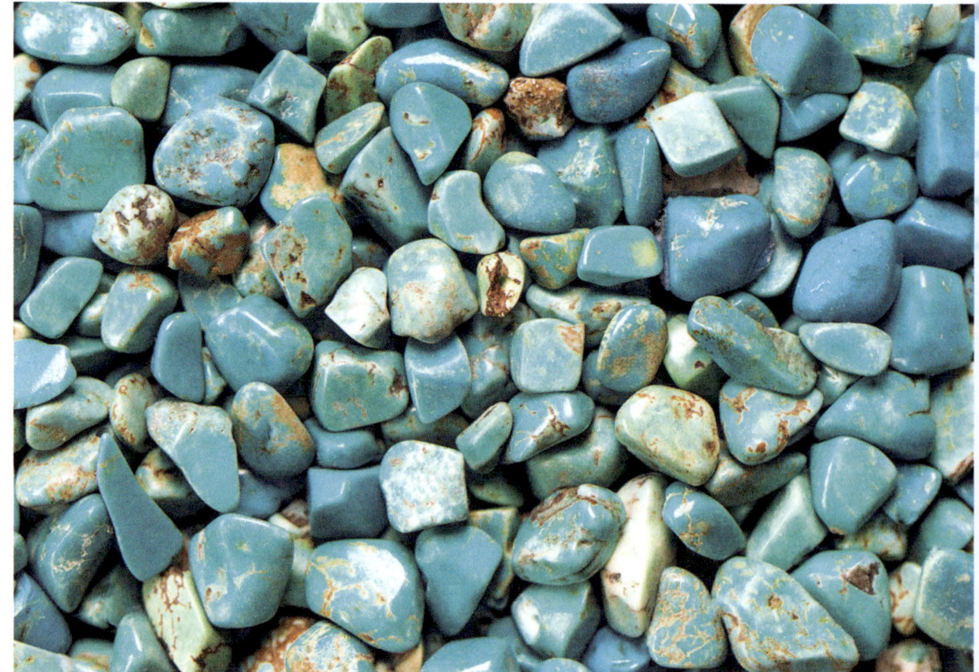

Turquoise

TO MAKE A CONNECTION

Speak up and make yourself heard. Turquoise supports clear and confident communication – it will help you be open and honest with those around you. It will give you the courage to honestly share your opinions, and if you're a bit shy it will anoint you with the bravery you need to shine in social situations.

HOW TO USE IT

Turquoise activates the throat chakra, your centre of communication and expression. So the best place to keep a turquoise stone is close to your throat on a pendant. Wear it when you need to speak in public, or if you need to have a tricky conversation.

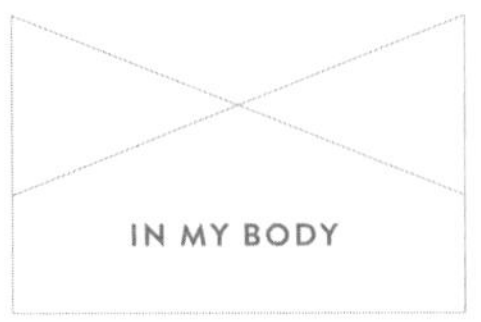

Breathwork to Speak Out

BREATH OF JOY

Breathe to awaken your system, get your energy flowing and give voice to your spirit.

1.
Stand with your feet shoulder-width apart and parallel, knees slightly bent.

2.
Inhale one-third of your lung capacity and swing your arms up in front of your body, parallel to each other at shoulder level with palms facing upwards.

3.
Inhale to two-thirds capacity while stretching your arms to the side. Inhale fully and swing your arms parallel over your head.

4.
Exhale completely with an audible "ha!", bend the knees more deeply and sink into a standing squat. Repeat.

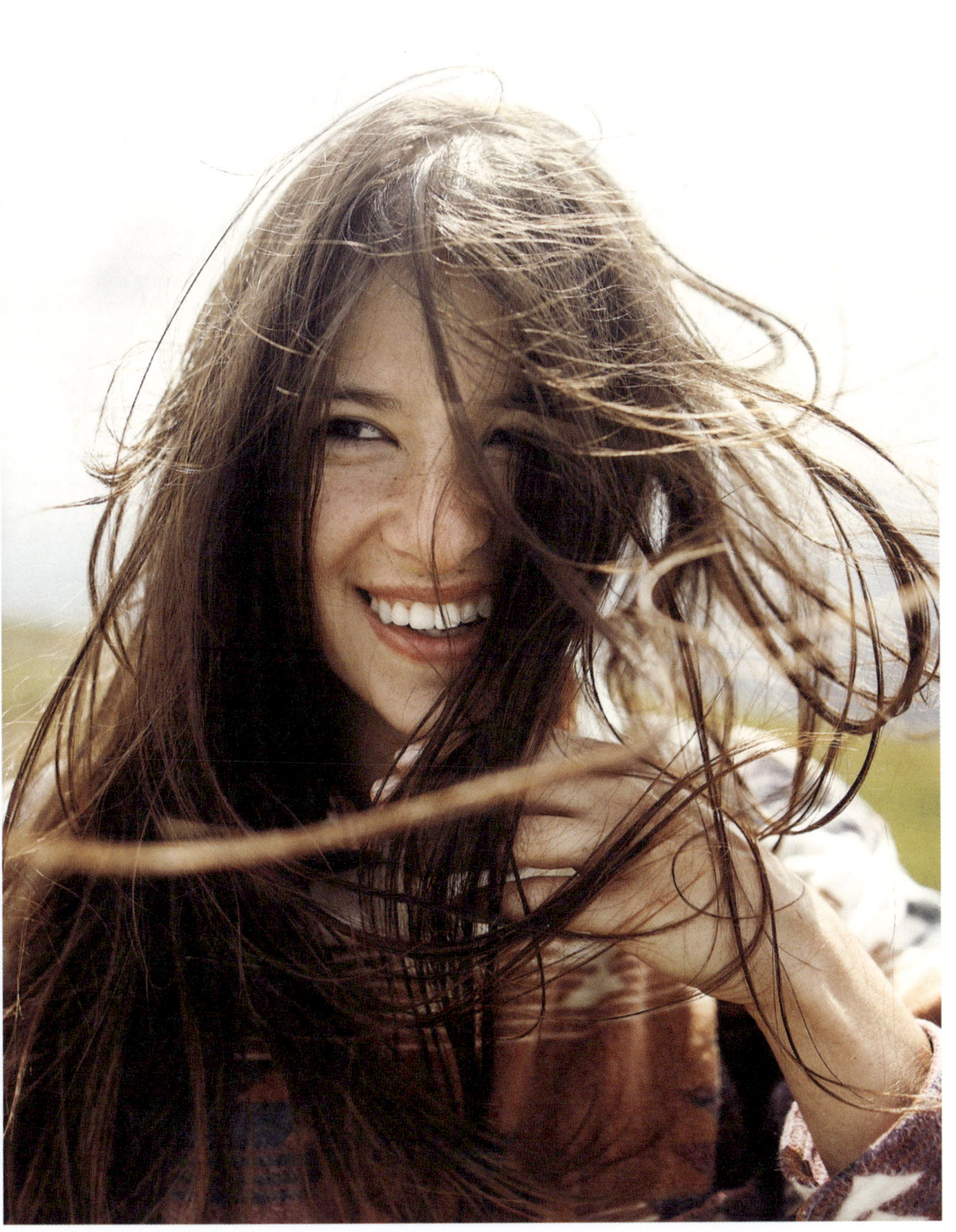

AFFIRMATION

I am loyal to my friends and they are loyal to me.

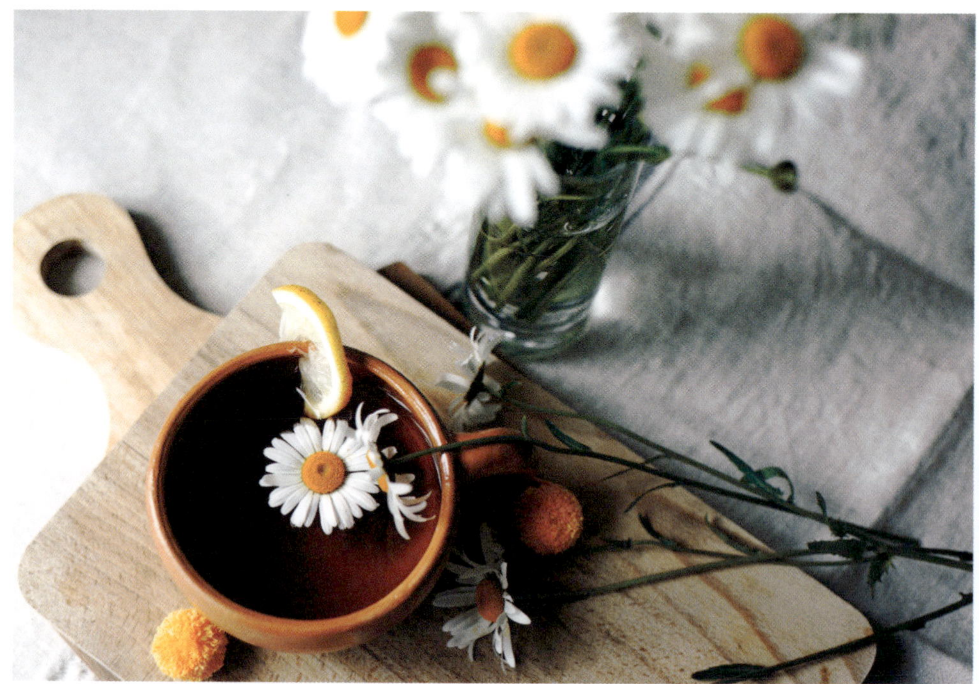

Chamomile

FOR FRIENDSHIP

Delicate yet resilient, chamomile is a neat metaphor for friendships – treat it with respect and it will give you joy and last forever.

Planting it is like having your most supportive confidante waiting at your window (or in your garden). It's one of the best herbs for friendship, luck, money and healing, also great for relaxing and soothing frazzled nerves.

HOW TO USE IT

Chamomile's superpower is as a tea. Place fresh or dried flowers in a cup of hot water, add honey if you like and sip slowly. Make a cup when a friend visits for a calming afternoon tea. Taken just before bed, it will lull you into a peaceful night's sleep.

Claddagh Ring

Two hands enclose a heart adorned with a crown, symbolising the bonds of friendship, love and loyalty.

There's a romantic story behind one of Ireland's most enduring symbols. Legend has it that a 17th-century Irish fisherman was kidnapped by pirates and sold into slavery in Algeria. His master taught him the craft of goldsmithing. Released after 14 years, he returned to Galway where he found that his sweetheart had waited for his return.

He gave her the ring he designed while in captivity, with its heart of love, crown of loyalty and hands of friendship. And naturally, they got married.

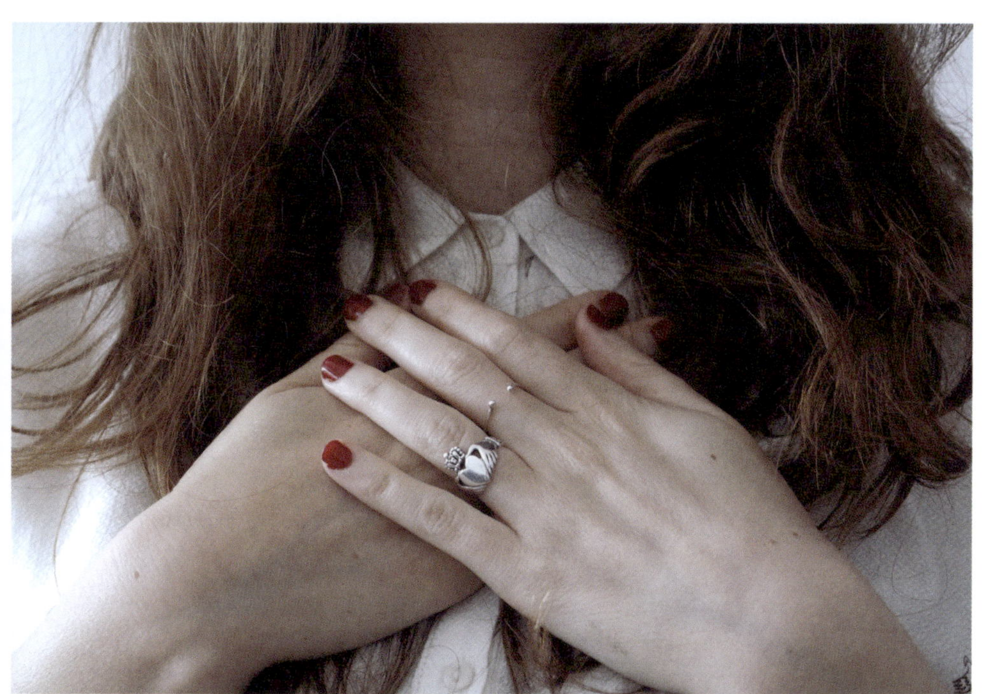

OTHER SYMBOLS OF LOYALTY

Dogs

Elephants

Swans

Knotted rope

The colour blue

Bamboo

Forget-me-nots

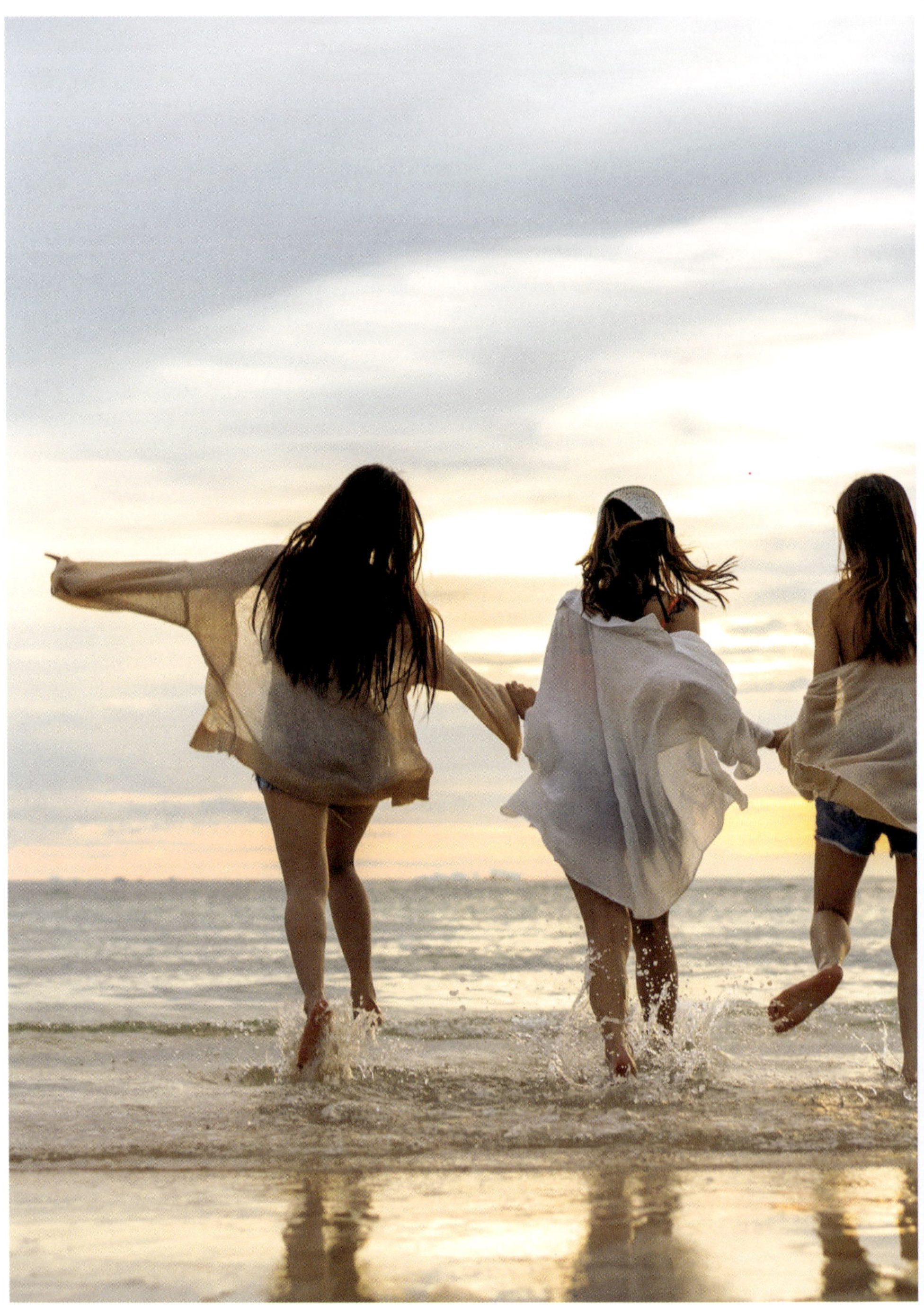

"BE WHO YOU ARE AND SAY WHAT YOU FEEL, BECAUSE THOSE WHO MIND DON'T MATTER AND THOSE WHO MATTER DON'T MIND."

— BERNARD BARUCH

CHAPTER TWO

Practise Empathy xx

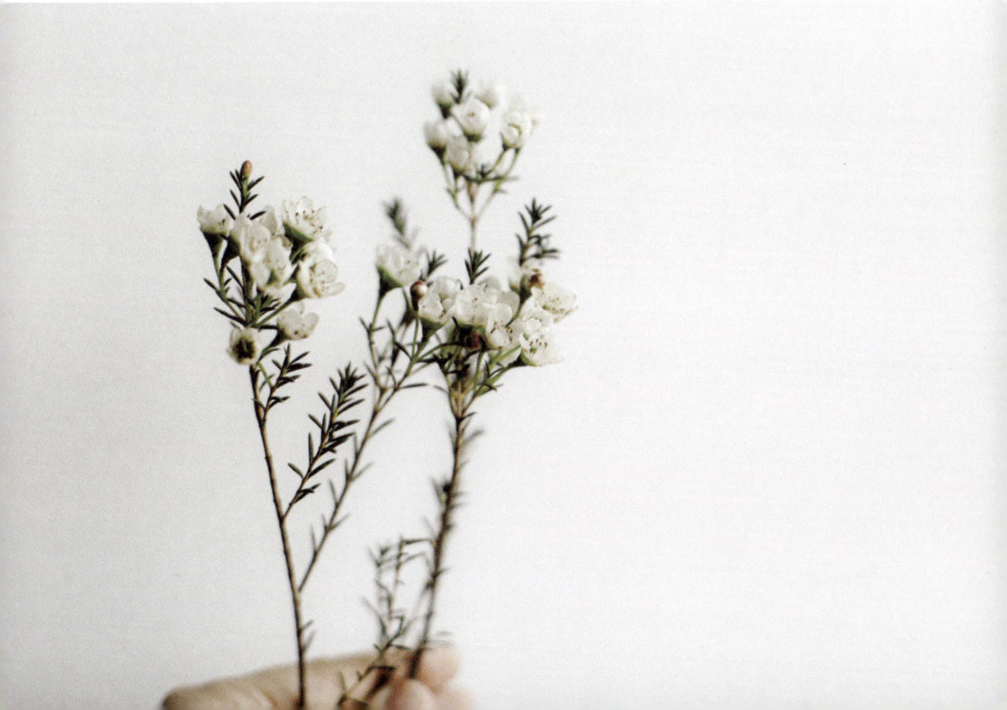

> “We are stronger when we listen, and smarter when we share.”
>
> RANIA AL ABDULLAH

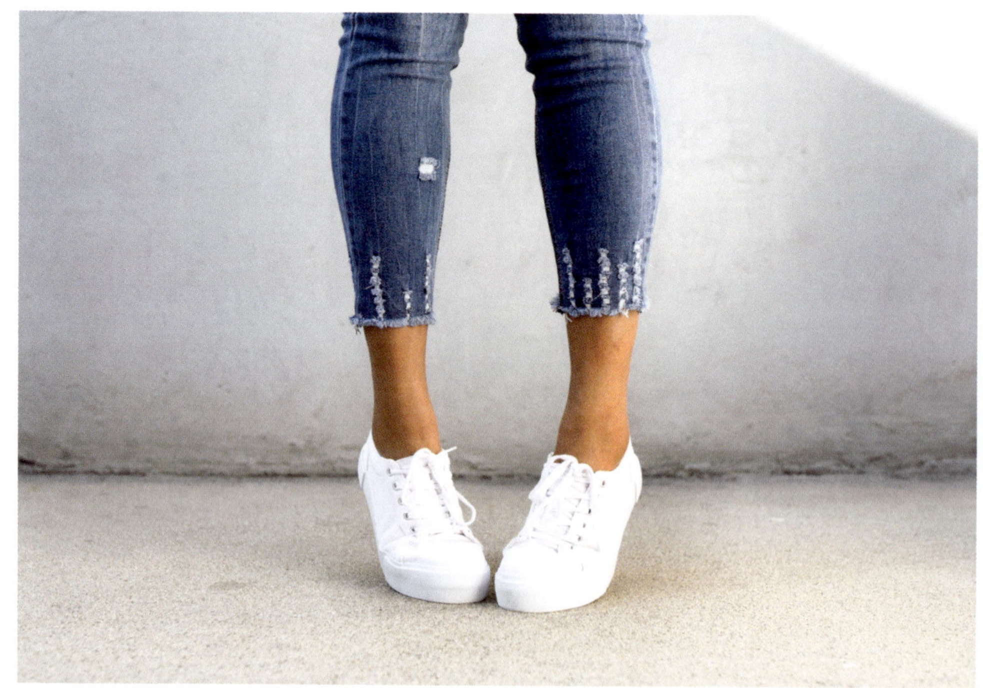

Other peoples' shoes

"You can't understand someone until you've walked a mile in their shoes."

You've probably heard the saying, but what does it mean? In a word, it's about empathy. Empathy is being able to share and understand someone else's emotions.

If we sense someone is feeling awkward, we encourage them to relax. If we feel someone is delighted, we share their joy. What we say, and how well we listen, is a marker of how good our empathy skills are.

Respectful listening is about tuning in to the other person to better understand who they are as a human being. We're all different. But as we open our ears to the struggles of others, we understand that they're also our struggles – feeling worthy, seeking purpose, just doing our best. And as a wonderful side-effect of empathy, we start to feel better about ourselves, too.

What empathy means to me

Use this section to explore the meaning of empathy. Create your own definition and consider what or who is important when you think about it. What does empathy mean in your life?

My definition of empathy is …

It makes me think of …

> “We rise by lifting others.”
>
> ROBERT INGERSOLL

I experience it when ...

Trading places

Empathy starts with imagination. Try this. Think of a tricky situation you are having with someone. Write down your thoughts and feelings about it. Then put yourself in the place of the other person. Write down the thoughts and feeling you think they may have.

The situation is ...

"You can only understand people if you feel them in yourself."

JOHN STEINBECK

I think and feel ...

The other person might think and feel ...

Now imagine a wise person (real or imagined) reading the two versions. What do you think their guidance would be?

The honesty challenge

Sharing your innermost feelings about something can bring a relationship to a new level. And when you're open and honest with yourself about your own feelings it's easier to listen with empathy, and to communicate openly with others.

Write four statements about things that you feel deeply about, using this formula:

"I feel ... about ... because ..."

I feel ...

I feel …

I feel …

I feel …

Imagine sharing these feelings with a particular person in your tribe. What do you think their response might be?

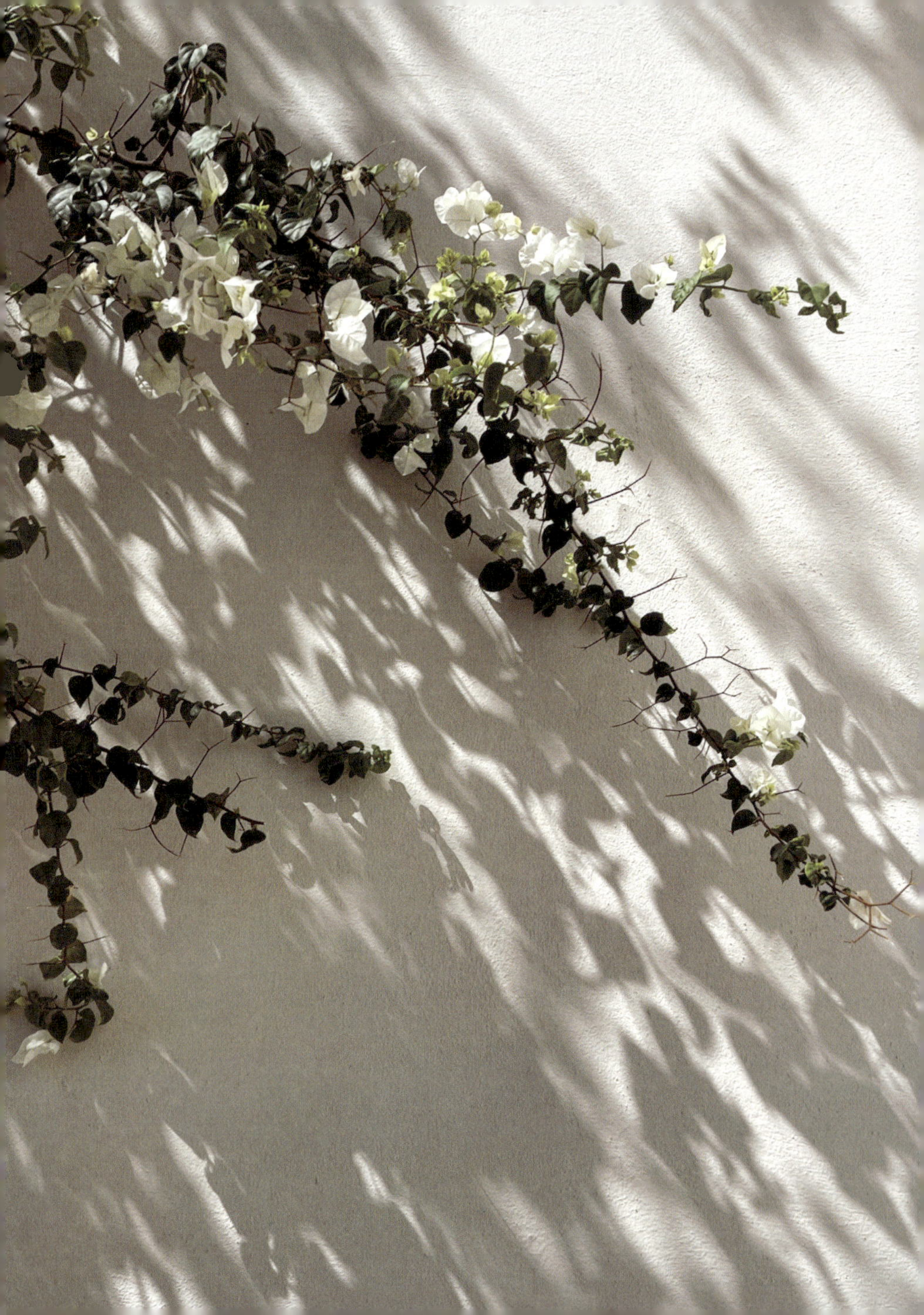

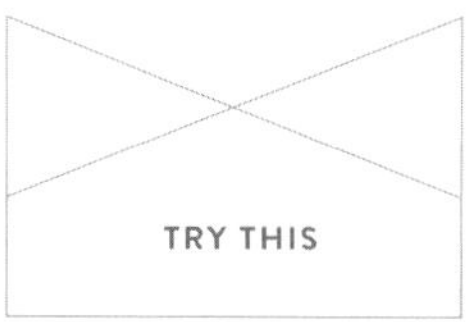

Loving Kindness Meditation

Send loving energy towards yourself and others to open your heart and give your empathy muscle a workout.

HOW TO DO IT

Find a quiet space and get comfortable. Create a mantra of caring for yourself and others (for example, "May I be happy, healthy and safe. May you be happy, healthy and safe").

Repeat the mantra in six stages: first direct it towards yourself, next towards someone special in your life, then towards a relative or friend, next towards someone you feel neutral about, then towards someone you dislike or have conflict with, and lastly, towards all beings.

While you repeat the mantra, visualise the caring wishes physically flying from you to the other people, connecting you to them with a link of goodwill.

Switch off, tune in

Mindful listening is the idea that we can ramp up our listening skills to create a deeper connection with another person. It means making contact with someone not only at a thought level but at a gut and emotional level too.

It's important to be undistracted – that means putting devices away and giving the person your full attention, with all your senses focused on what you are experiencing.

Listen closely to what they say. Put judgement aside and pay attention to their cues, trying to understand the message behind the words. Don't jump in with your own perspective. Let them express themselves fully. Don't be afraid to leave pauses to give them some time to reflect.

Consider what their experience or perspective might be. Be open and accepting of the possibility that it might be different to yours.

Respond meaningfully, connecting to what the other person just said. Meet them where they are, mentally and emotionally.

"We have two ears and one mouth, so we should listen more than we say."

– ZENO OF CITIUM

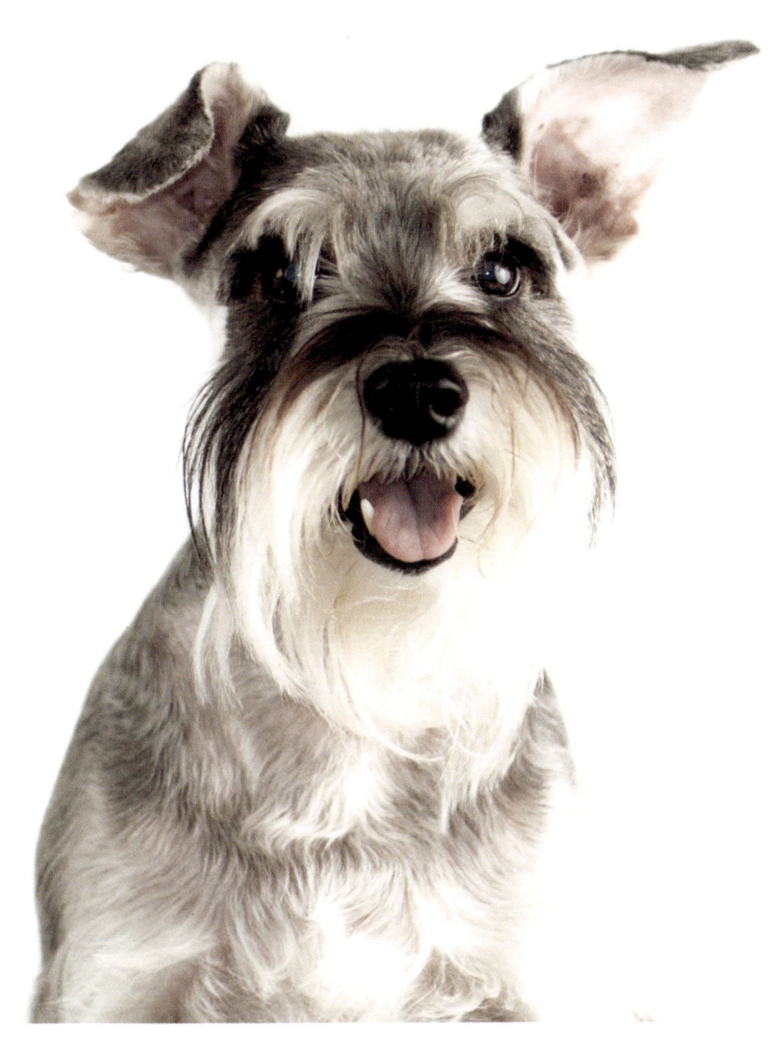

> **"First learn the meaning of what you say, and then speak."**
>
> — EPICTETUS

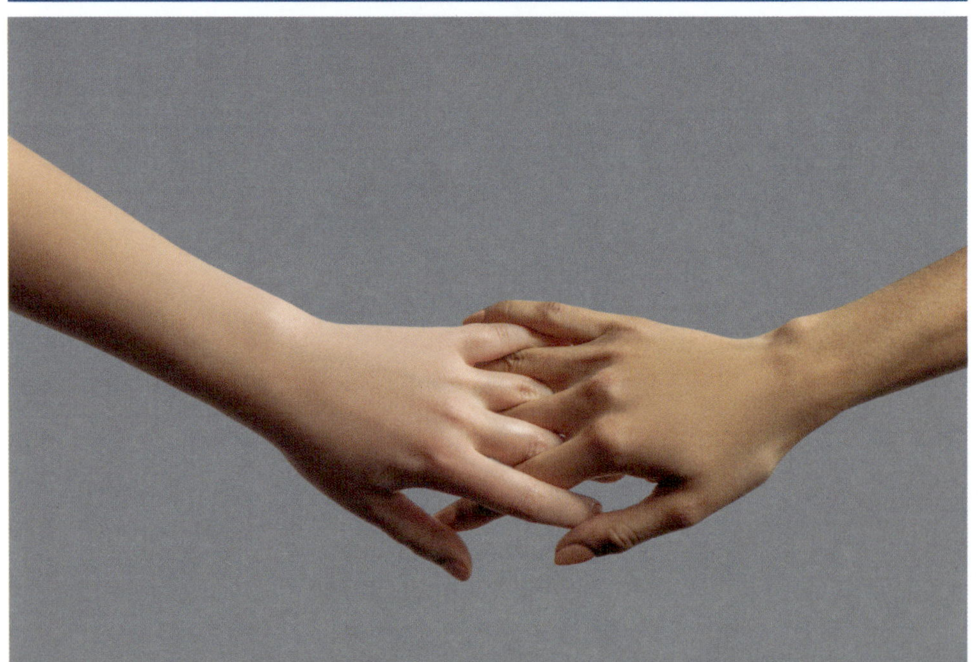

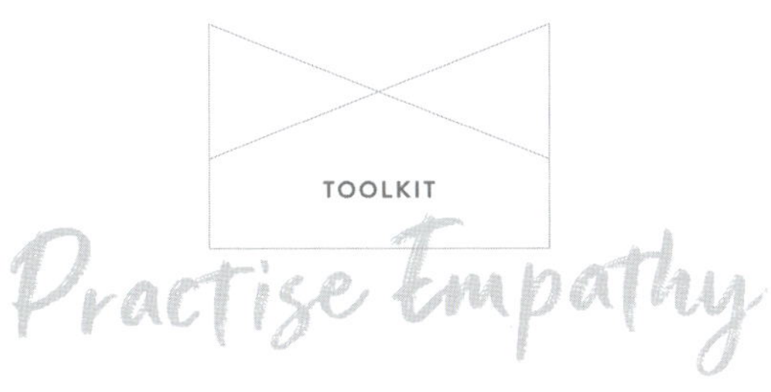

Speak your truth and truly listen:
Let elderflower tonic, lapis lazuli, shared breaths and the chatty dolphin guide you on your path.

AFFIRMATION

Today I practice the skill of being quiet.

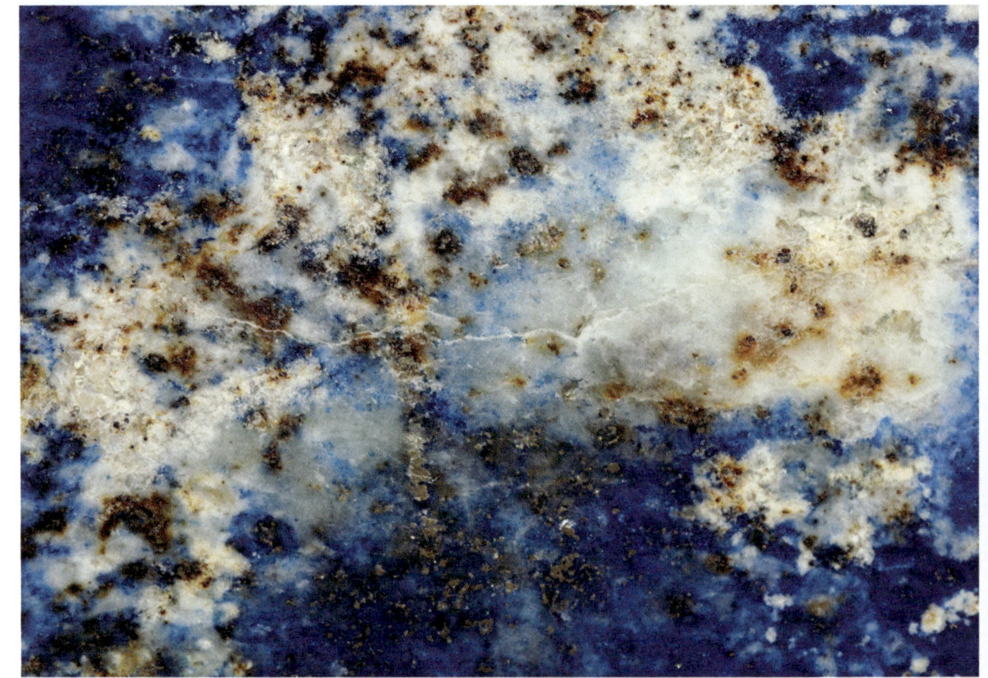

Lapis Lazuli

FOR ACTIVE LISTENING

Treasured for centuries as a stone of communication, lapis lazuli is one of the most powerful crystals for strengthening relationships, both platonic and romantic. It encourages positivity and commitment, and helps you communicate confidently, listen mindfully and be empathetic.

HOW TO USE IT

Lapis lazuli acts on the throat chakra to open the voice and the third eye chakra to deepen insight. Hold a lapis lazuli stone to your forehead (between the eyes) or the base of your throat to balance these chakras and connect more authentically.

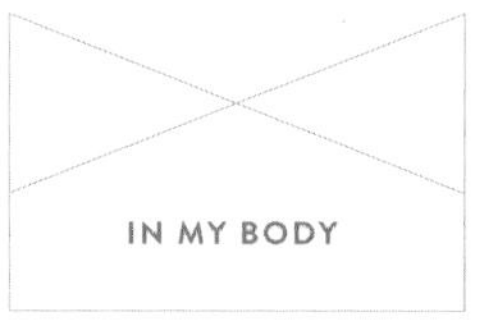

Breathwork for Empathy

CIRCULAR BREATHING TOGETHER

This intimate breathing exercise builds empathy and stimulates connection. Try it with someone you love.

1.
Lay, sit or stand facing one another. Take three deep, cleansing breaths simultaneously.

2.
Begin to breathe together until your breathing is in sync. Inhale and exhale together for a few rounds of breath.

3.
In the next round of breath wait until your partner exhales before you inhale. Then exhale while your partner inhales.

4.
Continue to breathe like this for as long as you can manage. If you fall out of sync, start again at step 2.

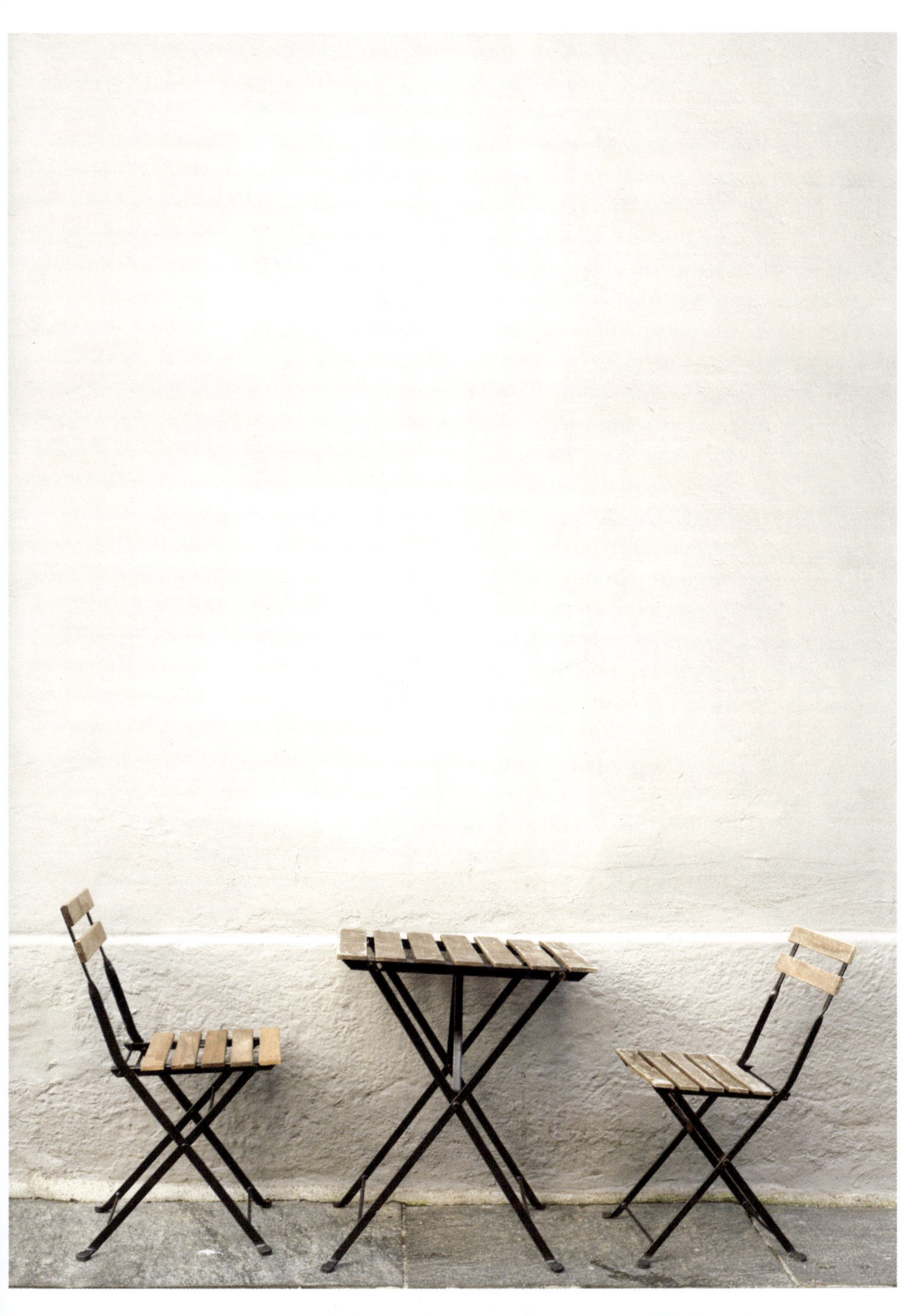

Elderflower and Honey Tea

An old-time herbal remedy with a pretty scent, elderflower soothes and opens the throat so communication can flow sweetly.

INGREDIENTS

¼ cup dried elderflowers

300ml boiling water

2 teaspoons honey

METHOD

Put the elderflowers in an infuser cup or teapot. Pour over the boiling water and steep for at least 10 minutes. Stir in the honey to taste.

Enjoy your tea in a comfortable and calming place, and let yourself rest in the moment.

AFFIRMATION

Today I practice the skill of being quiet.

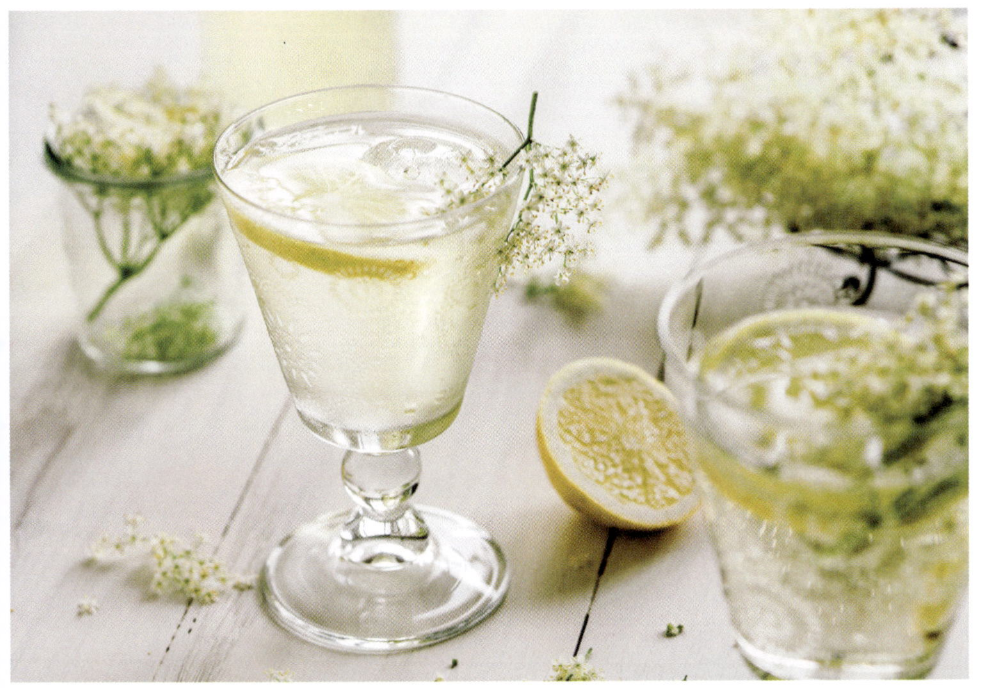

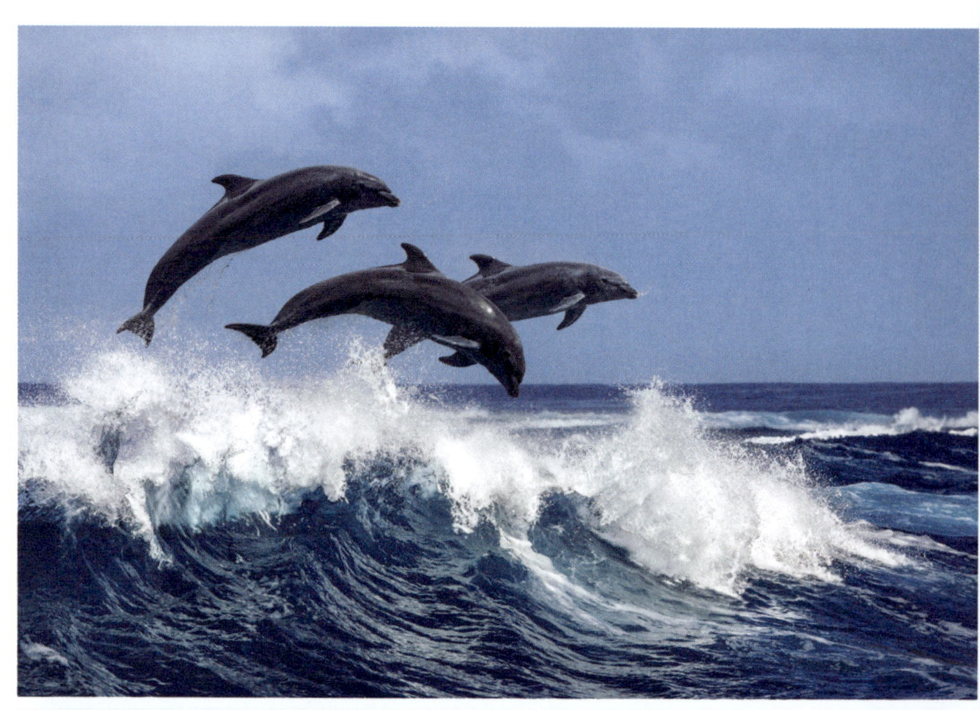

DOLPHIN BODY LANGUAGE

As well as their vocalised squawks, whistles, clicks and squeaks, dolphins use non-verbal communication like body postures, jaw claps, bubble blowing and fin caresses.

The Dolphin

A charismatic team player with a knack for saving those lost at sea, the dolphin symbolises community spirit and helping those in need.

Well-known for the squeaks and whistles they use to communicate with each other, dolphins also seem keen to widen their circle of friends. There are countless tales of dolphins making contact with water-bound humans through playful antics and even intervening to save people at risk of drowning. They seem to be always listening out for an opportunity to connect.

The dolphin is a reminder of the importance of communication. Be inspired by this aquatic empath to listen out for the messages that people send you, no matter how they arrive.

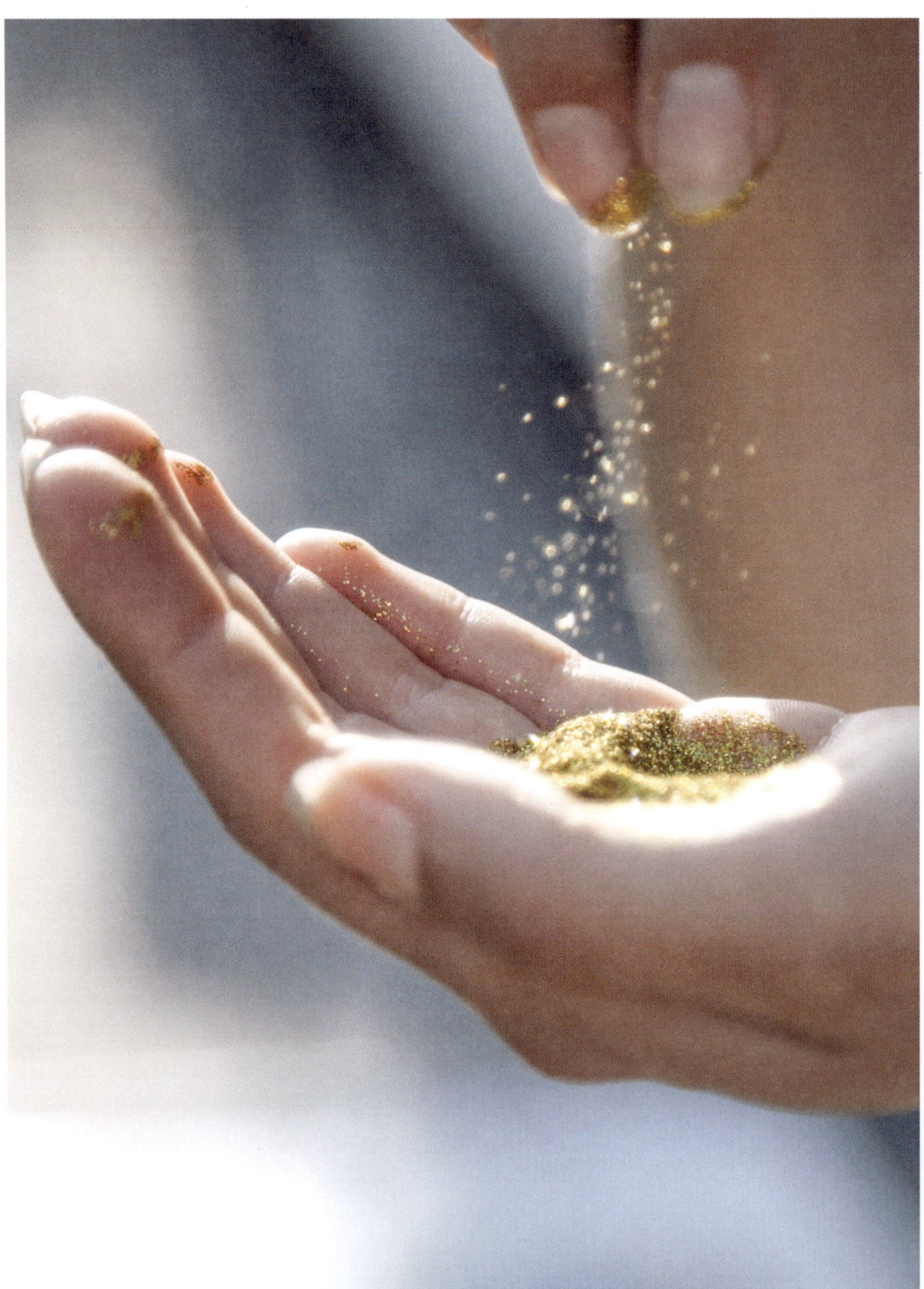

"IF SPEAKING IS SILVER,
THEN LISTENING IS GOLD."

— TURKISH PROVERB

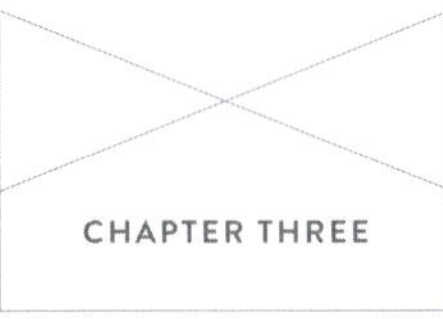

Own It xx

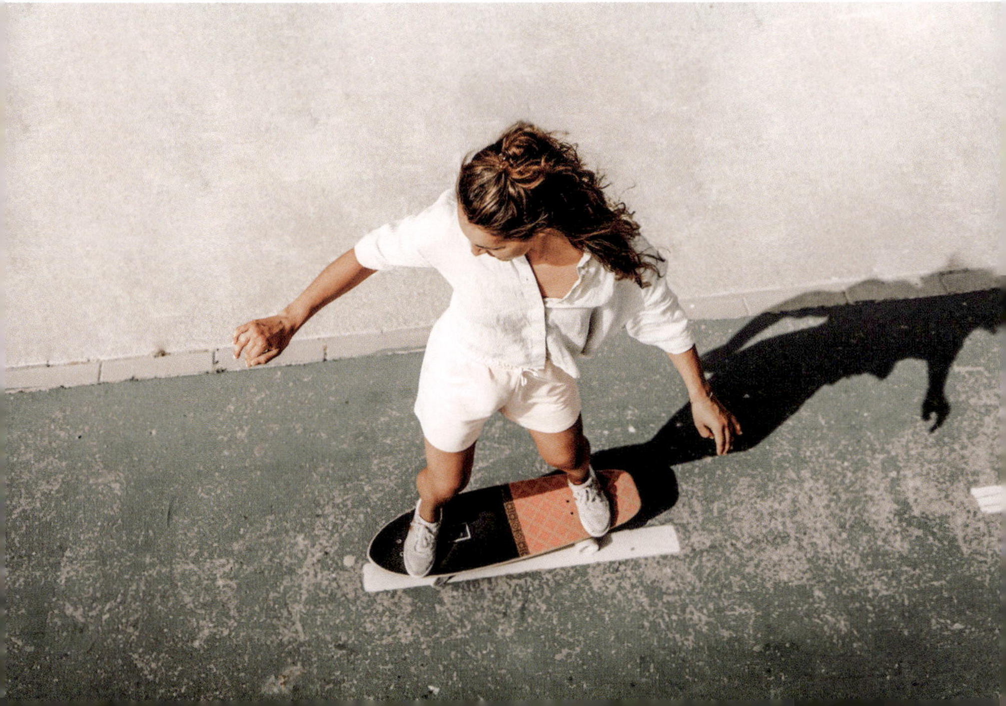

"I set boundaries not to offend you but to respect myself."

ANONYMOUS

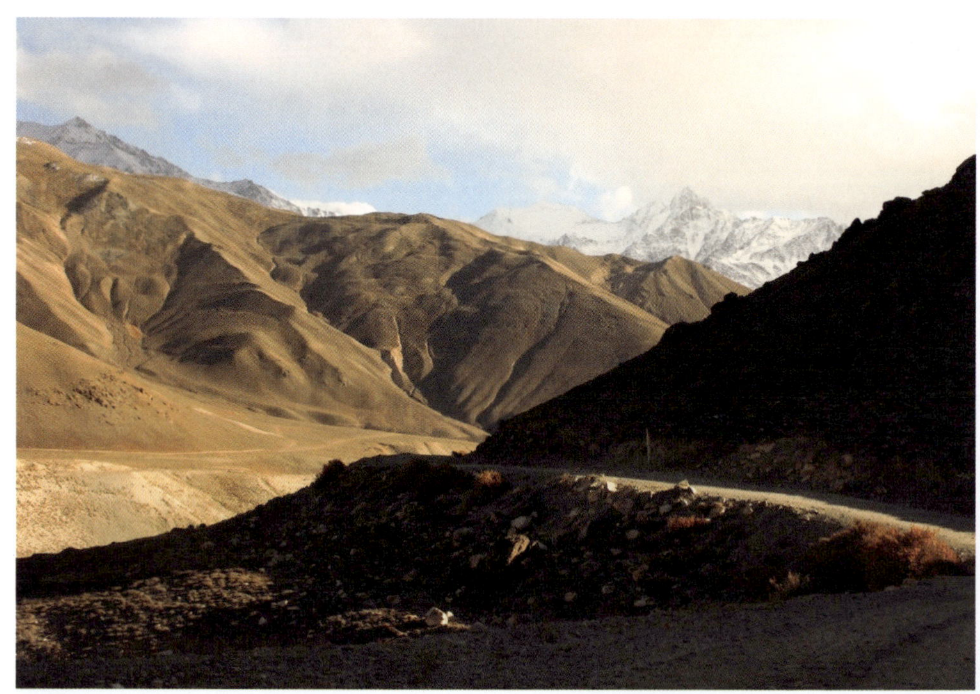

The frontiers of me

Do you know your boundaries?

Boundaries are about how emotionally close you let people get to you. They're where you draw the line in relationships, how much you're willing to give or take, what you say "yes" or "no" to. They apply to all relationships, but in some ways boundaries are really about your relationship with yourself. They help you honour *your* needs, goals, feelings and values.

Getting close to other people doesn't always feel totally comfortable. That's normal. Opening up and sharing our deepest thoughts and emotions can be scary. It takes vulnerability, and that's something that we usually try to avoid. But taking risks and putting ourselves out there is necessary to the feeling of belonging and joy we get from forming intimate relationships.

So own your boundaries, embrace your vulnerability and be brave. The results will be worth it.

What boundaries mean to me

Use this section to explore the meaning of boundaries. Create your own definition of the term, and consider what or who it brings up for you when you think about it. How does the idea of boundaries appear in your life?

My definition of boundaries is ...

"A boundary is not that at which something stops, but that from which something begins."

— MARTIN HEIDEGGER

It makes me think of ...

I experience it when ...

Dare greatly

The idea of "daring greatly" acknowledges that the feeling of vulnerability can lead us to act in certain ways, and encourages us to step outside it to go further, deepen connections and learn.

Think of a recent example where you felt vulnerable and use these pages to imagine how you could have reacted differently.

The situation was ...

"Vulnerability sounds like truth and feels like courage."

– BRENÉ BROWN

I felt vulnerable because ...

It made me feel ...

If I was "daring greatly", I would have ...

For example, think about how you could have asked someone for help instead of trying to work it out on your own.

Boundary hunting

Good relationships come from good communication. In intimate relationships, the only way you'll know your own and your partners' boundaries is to discuss them. To prepare, reflect on what your boundaries are in intimate relationships and write them down here. What are your wishes and expectations about how much time you spend together, displays of affection, sharing on social media, sex and intimacy?

Next you might write the questions you want to ask your partner about their boundaries.

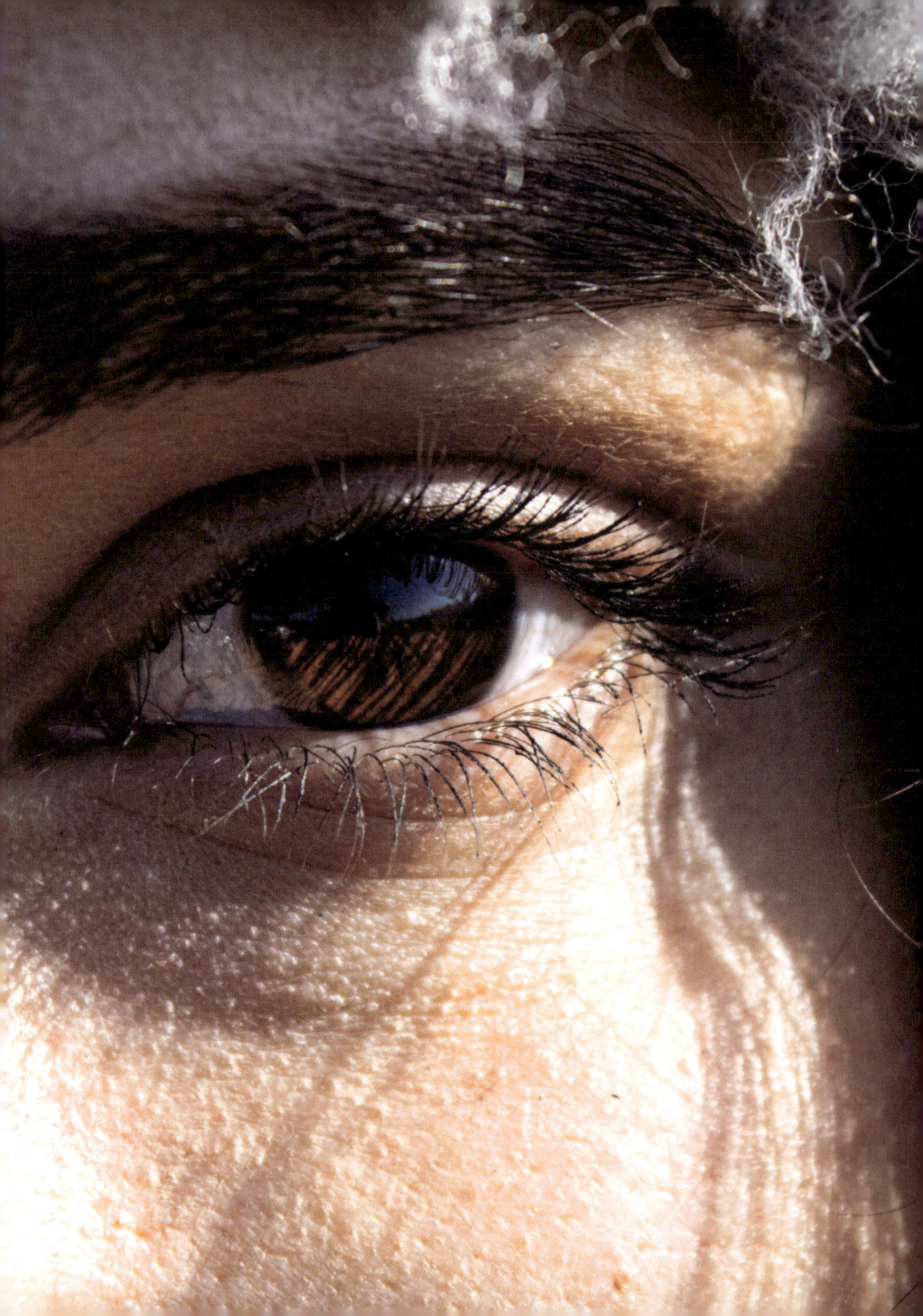

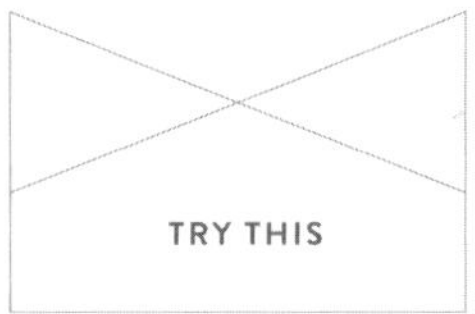

Perform an Eye-Gazing Ritual

There's a reason we call the eyes the windows to the soul. When we want to know how someone is feeling, we read their eyes.

Eye-gazing rituals are practised in Tantric and Buddhist traditions to deepen connections with other people and the Universe. Performing this ritual lets you explore what it feels like to truly see and be seen.

HOW TO DO IT

Sit in a comfortable position facing your partner. Hold hands, or place them on each other's knees. Set a timer and take a few deep breaths. Connect with their gaze, left eye to left eye. Keep breathing deeply and make your gaze soft.

Resist the urge to look away; allow thoughts and emotions to float by. Break your gaze gently when the timer sounds.

Feelings before words

When it comes to communication, what you say is often less important than how you say it.

Body language, facial expressions, eye contact, tone of voice – these things can speak more loudly than words. In tricky or challenging conversations, they can undermine communication and even create conflict. So how do we control that?

"Positive attunement" is the idea of tuning into the emotional state of another person. It happens by cultivating a real interest in and care for the other person. If you change your emotional state to one of attunement, your nonverbal language – as well as your words – will change.

So focus on the feeling of connection, rather than the message you want to deliver. Adopt the attitude that no matter whether you agree or not, you love and value the other person. And you'll find that communication becomes a whole lot smoother.

"Intimacy is the capacity to be rather weird with someone – and finding that that's OK with them."

ALAIN DE BOTTON

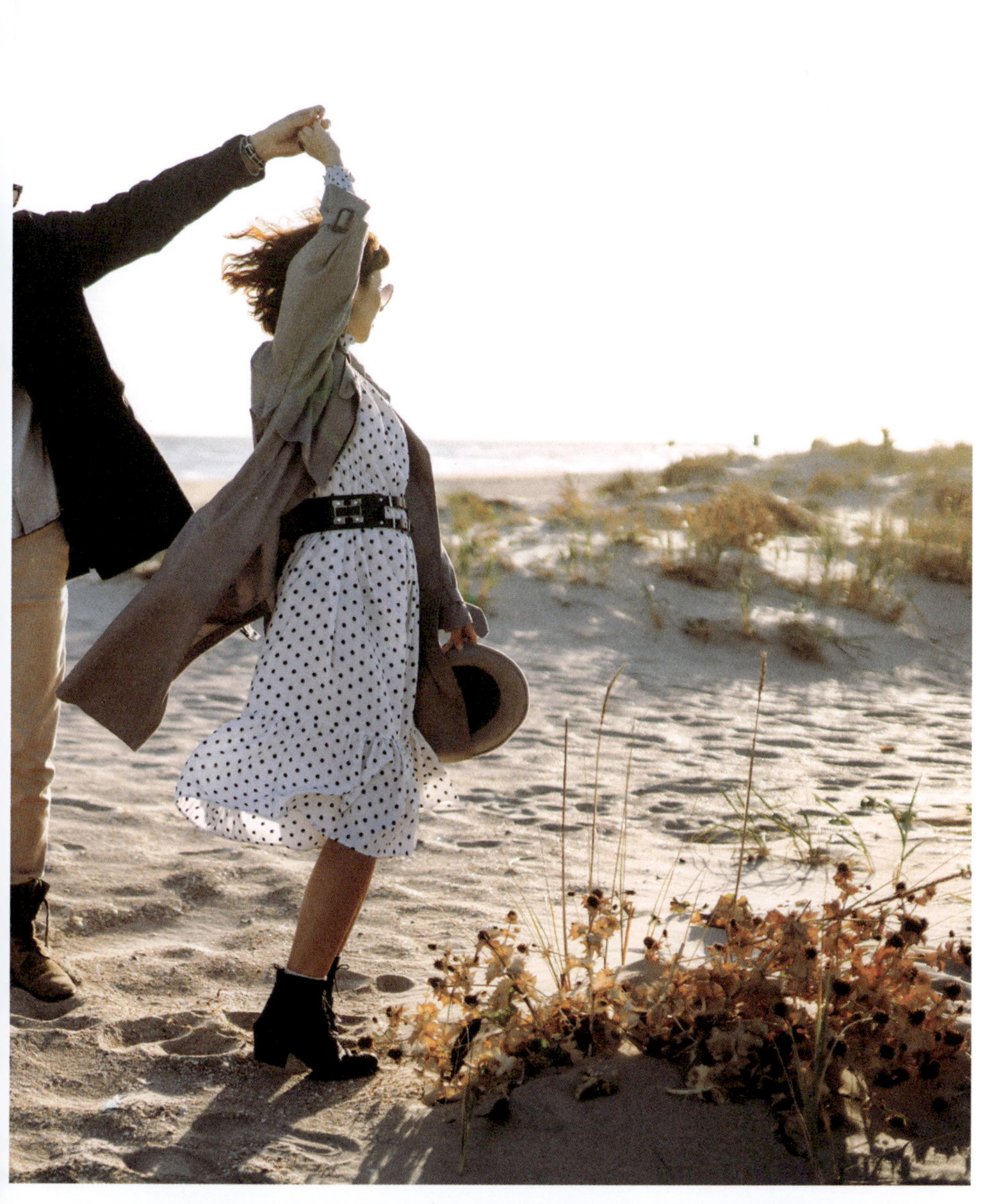

“Walls keep everybody out. Boundaries teach them where the door is.”

— MARK GROVES

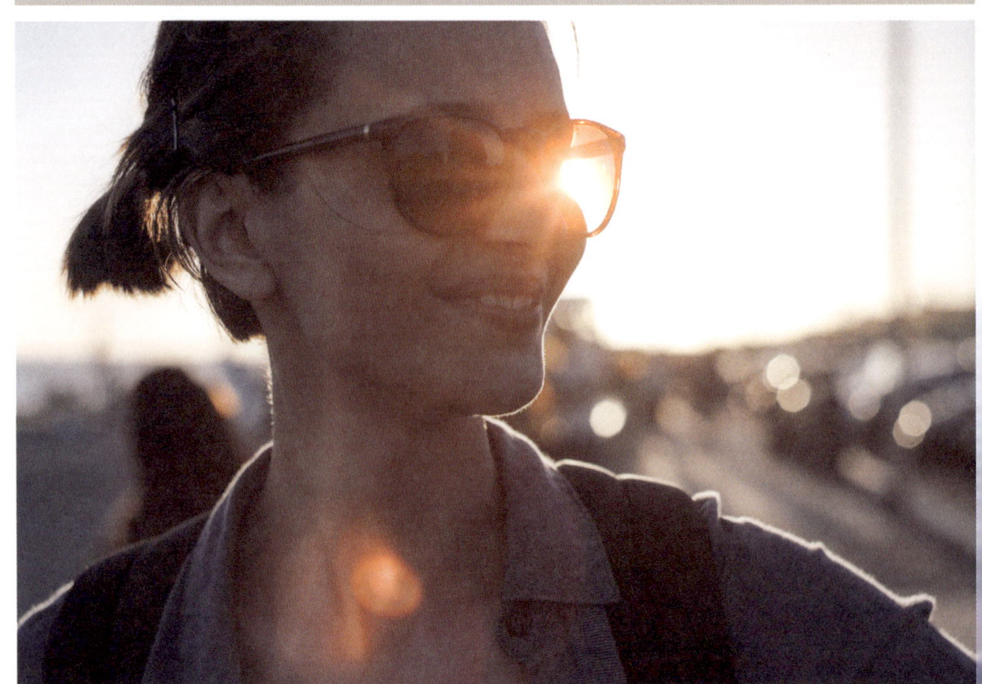

TOOLKIT

Own It

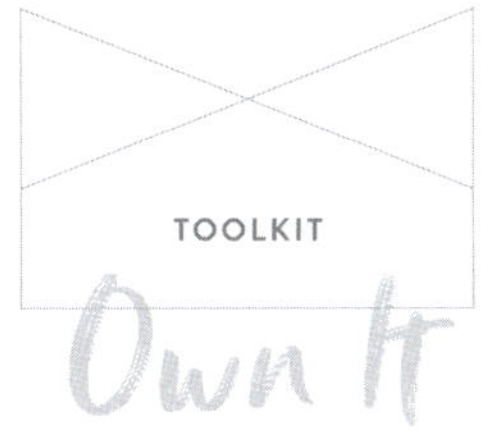

Be strong and stand your ground with support from victorious breathing, a gold-glinting mineral, an ancient herb and a fearless spirit guide.

AFFIRMATION

I can respect the feelings of others and still honour my own.

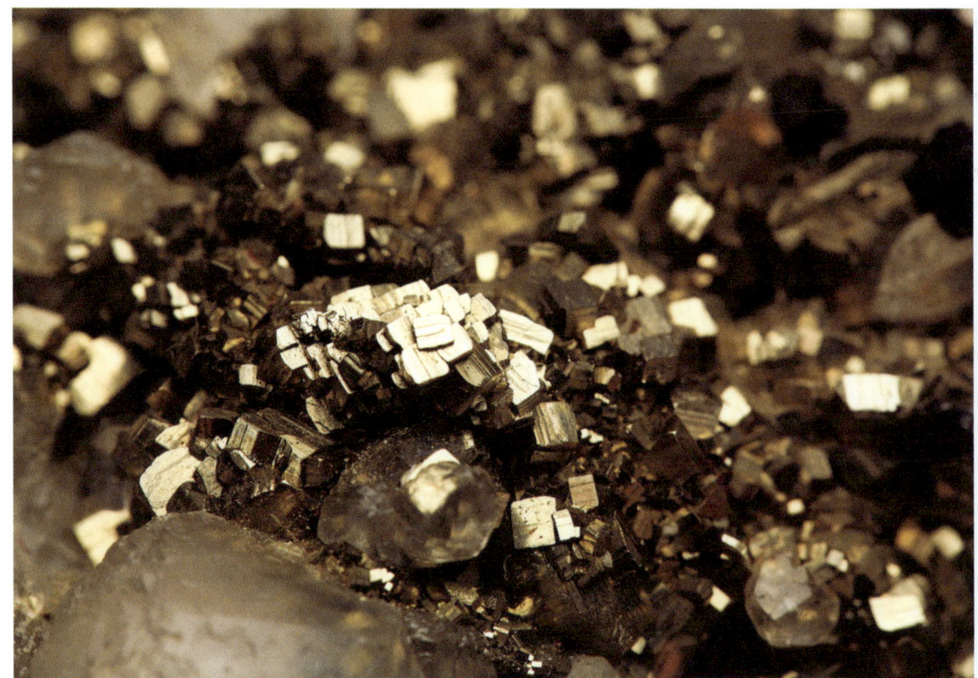

Pyrite

FOR STRENGTH AND PROTECTION

Commonly known as "fool's gold" because of its resemblance to the precious metal, pyrite is no phony when it comes to emotional power. It's all about keeping you strong and free from the shackles of control. It encourages leadership, inviting you to step into your potential – your self-awareness will prop you up.

HOW TO USE IT

Worn close to the skin, pyrite acts as an amulet or talisman, nourishing the body with its healing energy and protecting you from toxic energy. Wear a pyrite bracelet to remind you when to stand up for yourself and say "no".

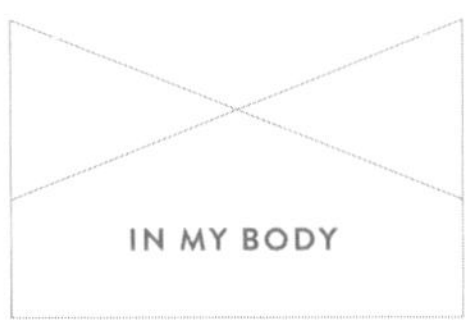

Victory Breaths

UJJAYI BREATHING

"Victorious breath" or "ocean breathing" creates a hypnotic sound that gathers your personal power and centres intention in your body.

1.
Lie on your back with a pillow under your head or knees.

2.
Breathe with your mouth closed, constricting your throat so your breath makes a rushing noise in and out, like the deep almost-snores of near sleep.

3.
Breathe into your belly, making your inhales and exhales equally long.

4.
Focus on the sound of your breath and how your body feels as you inhale. Be reminded of your internal power.

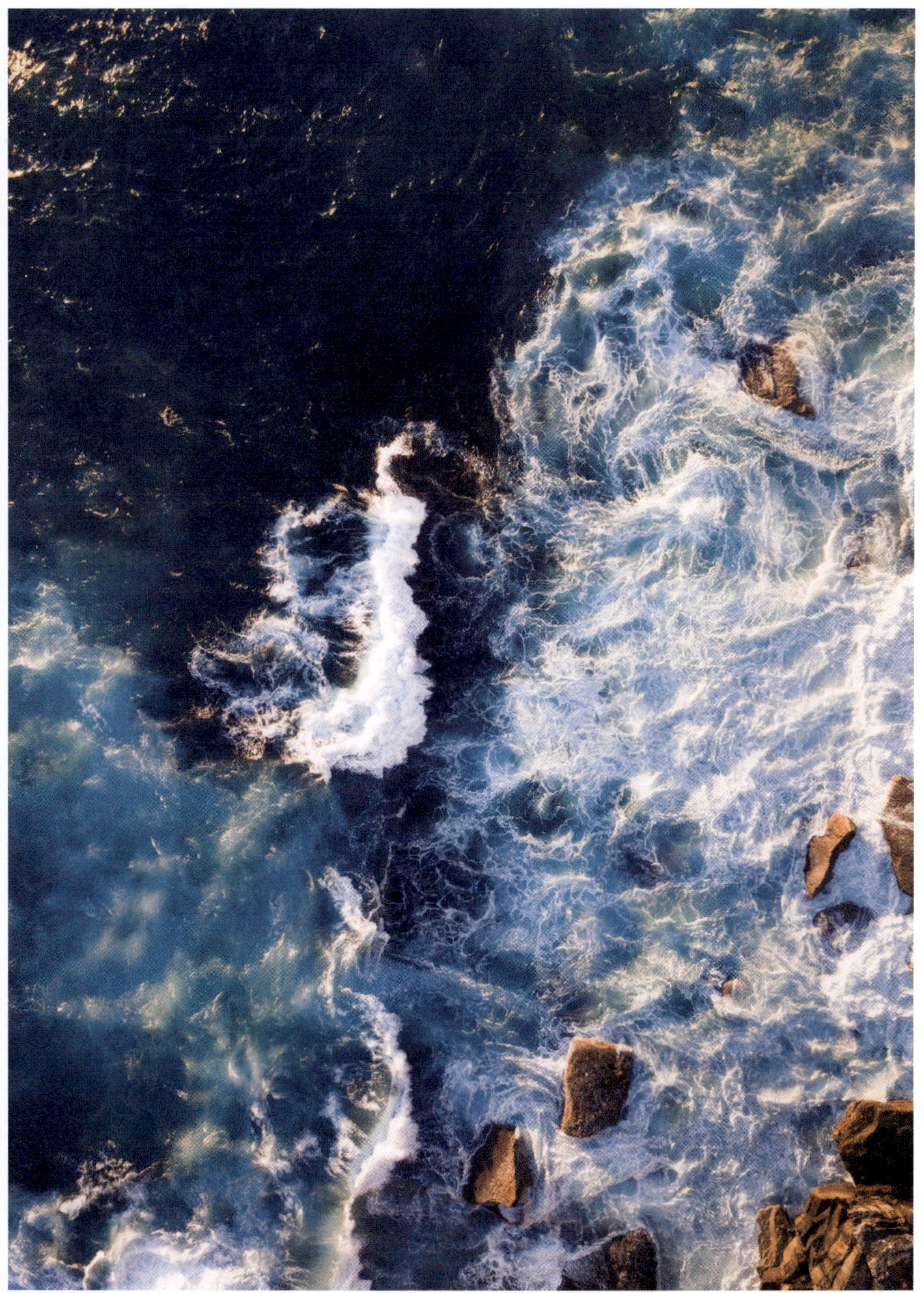

AFFIRMATION

I am allowed to say "no".

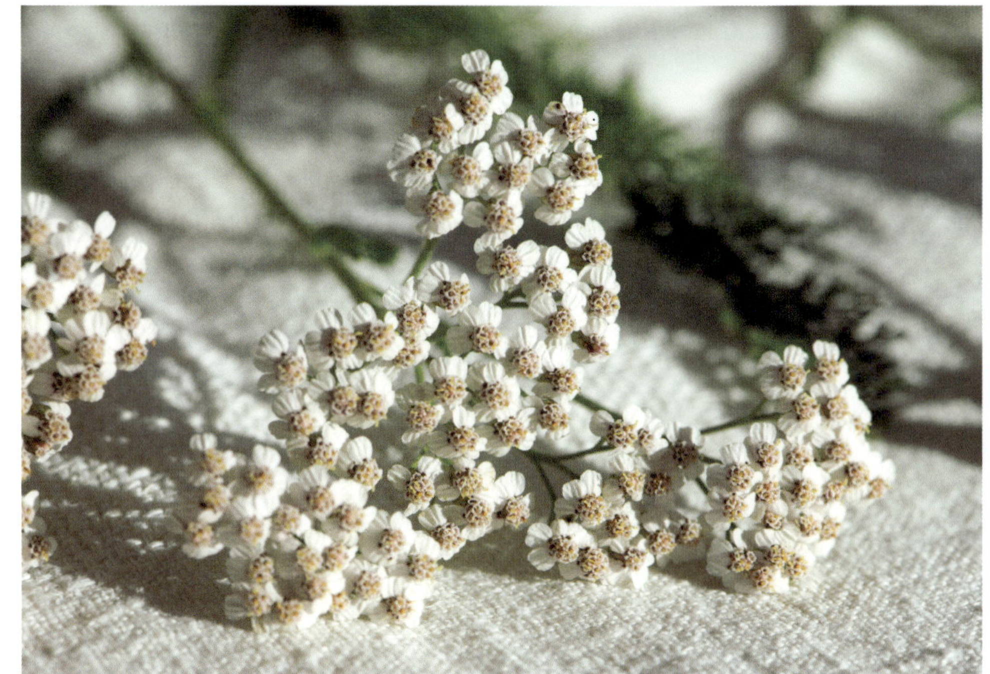

Yarrow

FOR STANDING YOUR GROUND

Yarrow has been used as a medicinal herb for centuries in many world cultures. It's most famous for its ability to stem bleeding and prevent infection, but it's also the patron plant of highly sensitive people. Yarrow helps us keep our boundaries strong, empowering our energetic field to form a protective bubble.

HOW TO USE IT

Make yarrow tea by adding a teaspoon of dried yarrow flower to a cup of boiling water, steeping for 30 minutes, then straining. Or get some yarrow essential oil to add to your diffuser – its herbaceous, slightly floral aroma soothes stress and lifts the mood.

The Wolf

Symbolising both a commitment to community and a desire for freedom, the wolf teaches us to stand our ground and make our position known.

The wolf is a complex beast. Both savage predator and loyal pack member, he has multiple personalities – menacing and dangerous in countless folk tales, revered by Native Americans as a pathfinder and loyal friend.

Wolves are social animals who thrive in well-structured societies. Despite their fierce reputation they go out of their way to avoid fights – but when they want to stave off an attacker, they know how to stand their ground. The wolf calls you to mark your territory clearly, fight your corner and stand up for your truth.

The wolf also symbolises animal instincts. As a spiritual guide, the wolf reminds us to go where our gut is telling us. When you're drawn to the wolf, listen carefully to what your intuition is saying.

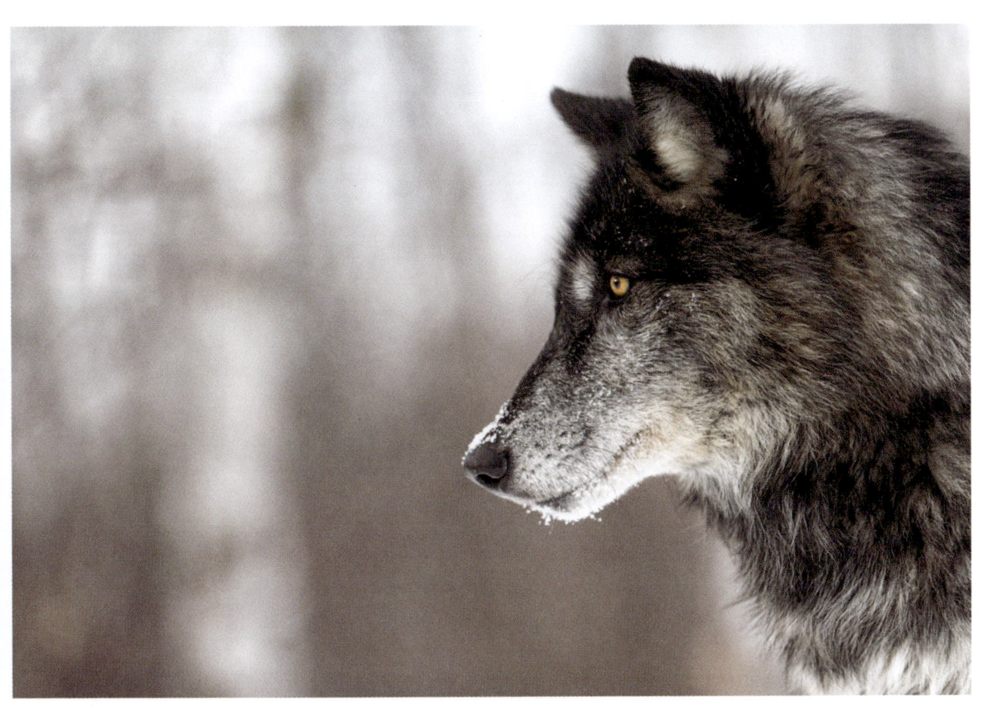

WOLF FAMILY LIFE

Wolves are devoted to family. They mate for life, educate their young, take care of their injured and live in extended family packs. They care for each other as individuals and there is even evidence that they grieve the loss of pack members.

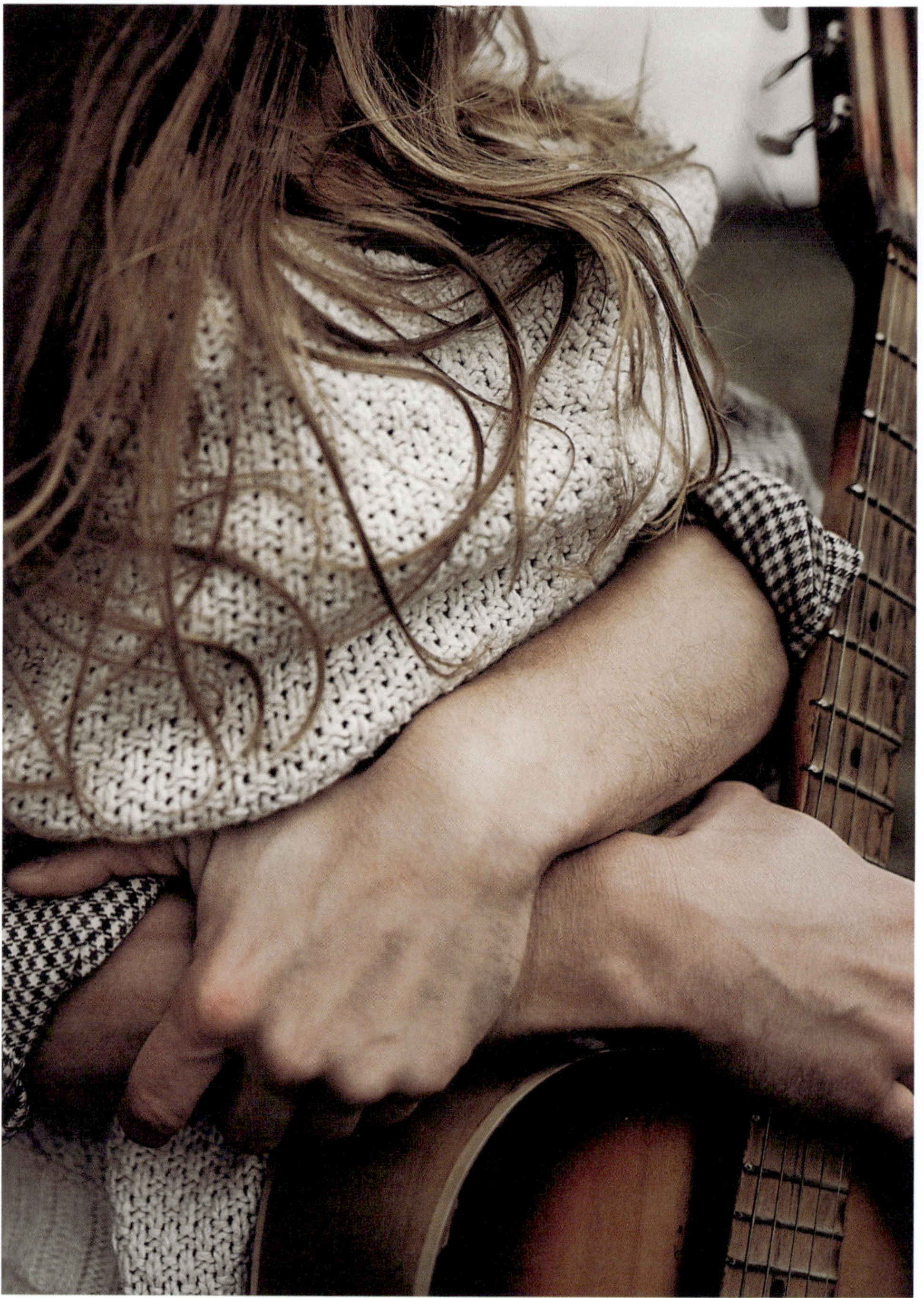

“VULNERABILITY IS THE ESSENCE OF CONNECTION AND CONNECTION IS THE ESSENCE OF EXISTENCE.”

— LEO CHRISTOPHER

CHAPTER FOUR

Connect Deeply xx

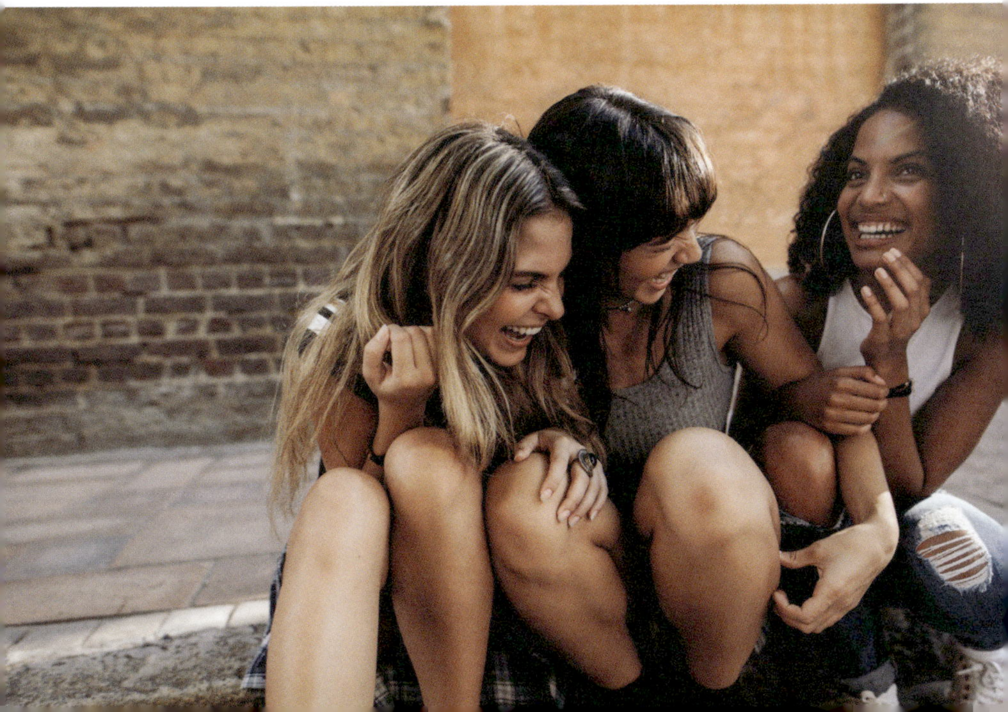

“Happiness is only real when shared.”

CHRISTOPHER MCCANDLESS

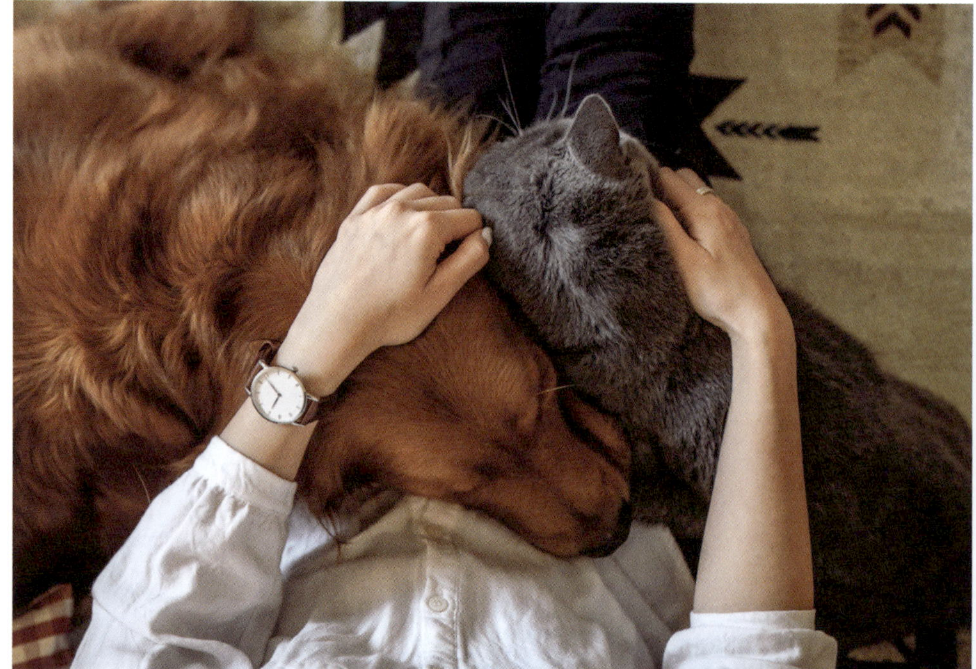

Hold on tight

Have you ever had the sensation of feeling alone in a room full of people? Even people with a wide social network can have feelings of isolation and loneliness. If you often have that sensation of disconnection, it might mean that your relationships lack intimacy.

When was the last time you had a truly deep and meaningful conversation with someone? Sharing your innermost thoughts, feelings, doubts and joys is one way to establish stronger bonds. Another is sharing passions, doing things together that you both enjoy.

Sometimes we forget to treasure what we have – we feel lonely because we've lost sight of how well supported we are. Make sure you acknowledge and honour your relationships by letting yourself feel a sense of gratitude for the people around you.

And don't forget that we build intimacy by sharing happy moments too – celebrations and good times create happy memories, a stock of positive thoughts we can revisit when we feel alone.

What intimacy means to me

Use this section to explore the meaning of intimacy. Create your own definition of intimate connection and consider what or who is important when you think about it. How do you experience it in your life?

My definition of intimacy is ...

"Only a life lived for others is a life worthwhile."

ALBERT EINSTEIN

It makes me think of ...

I experience it when ...

A meaningful moment

Think of a time when you felt a strong bond with someone in your life. What was the experience you had with this person where you felt especially close and connected to them? It could have been a time you had a meaningful conversation, gave or received support, experienced loss or success with them, or witnessed an historic moment together. Describe the ways this experience made you feel close and connected to the other person.

The experience where I felt this type of connection was …

It made me feel ...

I treasure you because ...

Choose five people. For each person write down one reason that you are grateful to have this person in your life. It might be a specific experience or an ongoing reason, a big thing or a small thing. What is it about this person that you value and hold dear?

I treasure

because ...

I treasure

because ...

"Enjoy the little things, for one day you may look back and realise they were the big things."

ROBERT BRAULT

I treasure

because ...

I treasure

because ...

I treasure

because ...

Now think about telling each of these people what you have written down here. Sharing your gratitude is a sure way to deepen your connection.

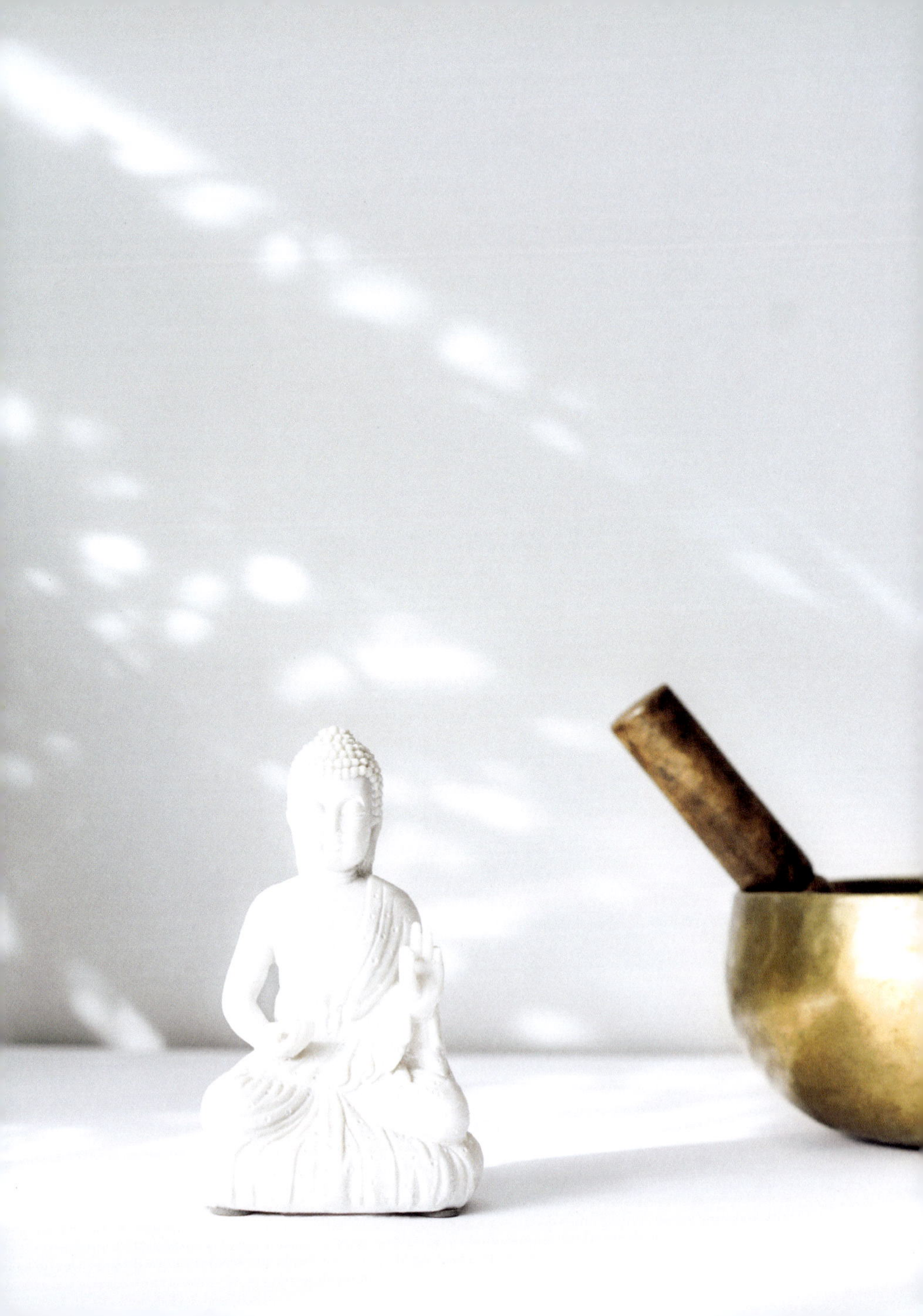

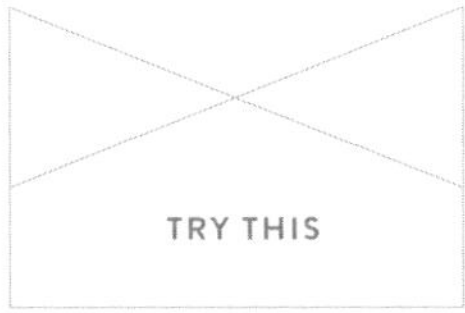

Start a Meditation Routine

It might seem strange, but sitting quietly on your own can deepen your connection with others. Yes, regular meditation can help develop a stronger sense of intimacy.

How? It makes us more accepting of our own flaws, so we're more forgiving of others. And it improves our ability to separate thoughts from emotions, making us less reactive so we're better able to weather relationship ups and downs.

HOW TO DO IT

In theory, nothing could be easier: All you need is a quiet place and a few minutes each day. But establishing a regular practice takes discipline, so you might like a helping hand. There are plenty of how-tos available online, and guided meditations on Spotify. Apps like Headspace or Calm give a step-by-step introduction.

Be the friend you want

Relationships have their own karma: You get out what you put in.

Make a point of catching up with your loved ones frequently. Be the instigator. It feels good. Arrange a regular get-together with family or friends, establish ongoing dates that are always in the calendar – a monthly dinner or weekly walk in the park.

Make sure you have all the important birthdays saved in your phone and set reminders early enough to buy a present or send a card (yes, a real cardboard one!)

Be the thoughtful friend that you want for yourself.

Hug. Get that feel-good oxytocin flowing.

Say "I love you" often. Or show it in your actions.

You'll find that it comes flowing back to you.

"Attention is the rarest and purest form of generosity."

– SIMONE WEIL

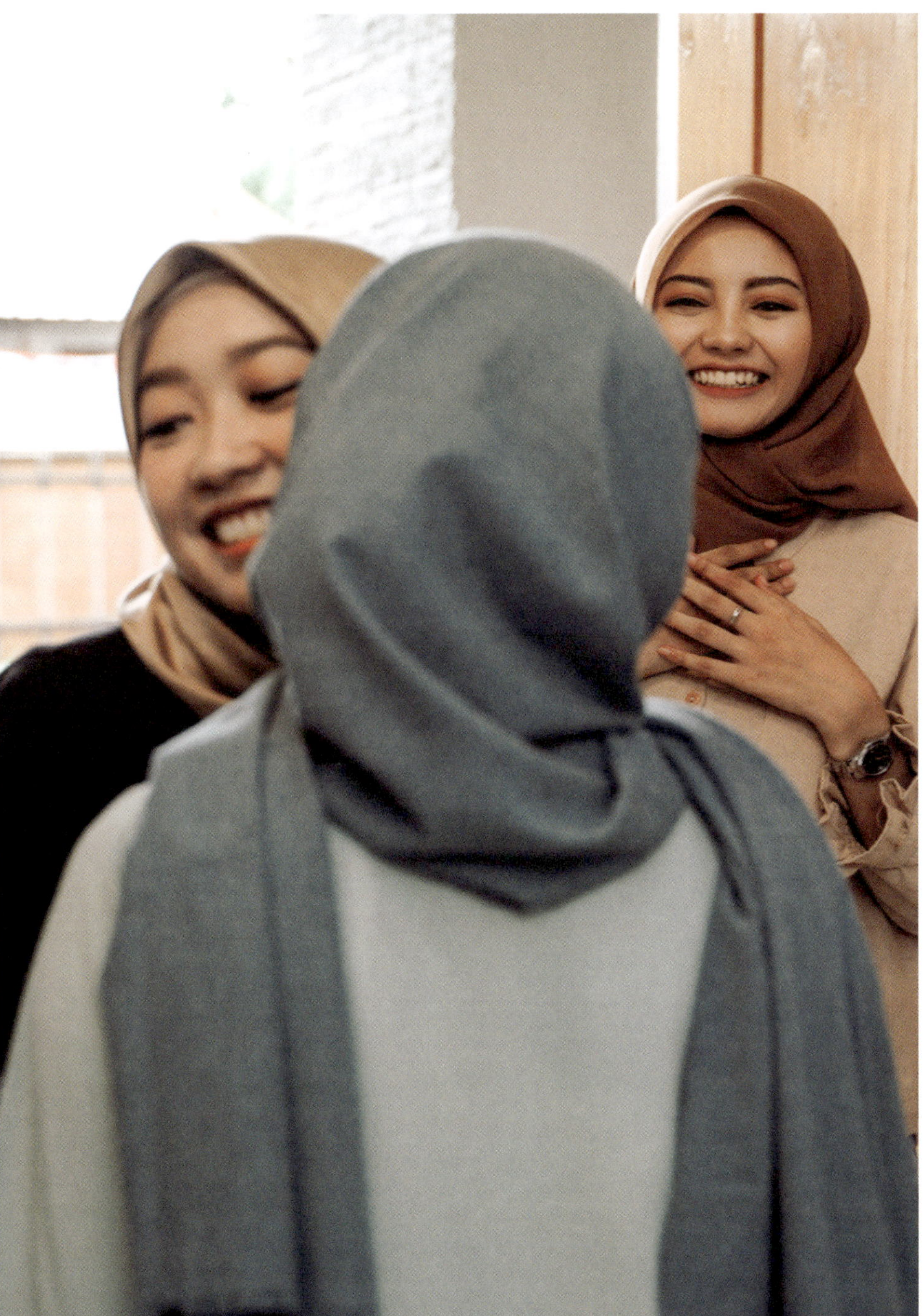

> "See the light in each other. Be the light for each other."
>
> — ANONYMOUS

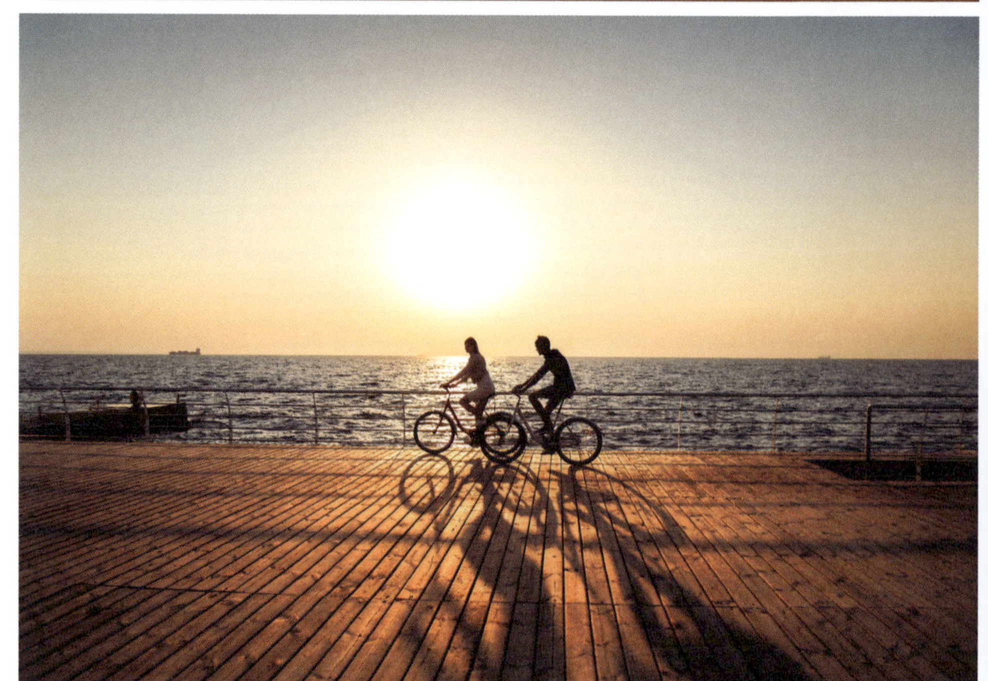

TOOLKIT

Connect Deeply

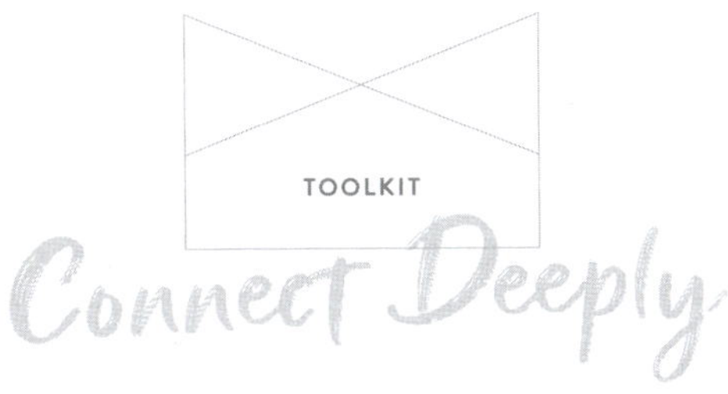

Nurture unconditional love and connection with precious emerald, luscious chocolate, a body-centred meditation and some help from a faithful companion.

AFFIRMATION

I am surrounded by love.

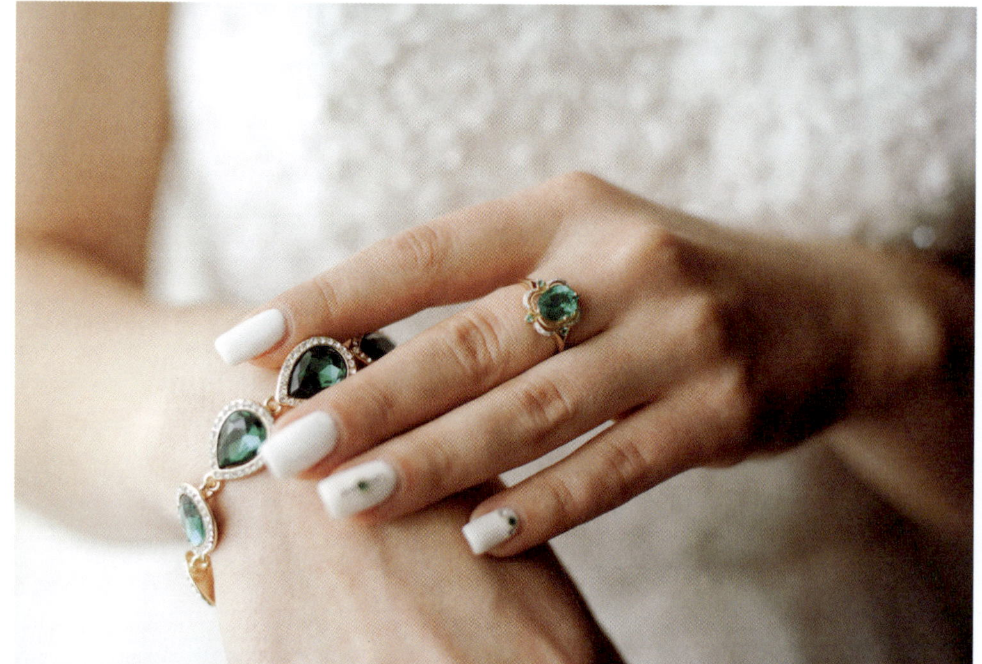

Emerald

FOR AUTHENTIC CONNECTION

Emerald is the stone of eternal love. It calls to the heart and clears out any weight or dark energy clogging up your emotions. With a sense of lightness comes a willingness to let in those you love and make an authentic connection. Emerald is a gem for deepening relationships, facing the fear of unveiling your true self and making a commitment.

HOW TO USE IT

This luscious gem's luminous properties, calming green hue and association with everlasting love make it a beautiful stone to give as a gift to someone special. Worn on a pulse point as a bracelet or ring, it sends healing, loving vibrations straight to the heart.

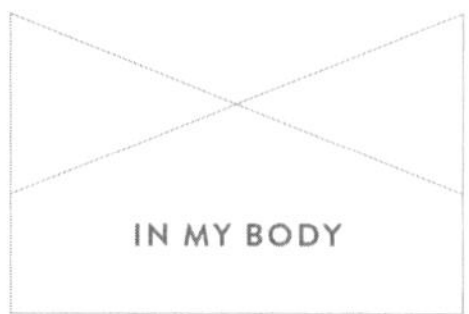

Meditation for Self-Connection

BODY SCAN MEDITATION

Do a deep listening session with your body to tune in to your authentic self.

1\.
Lie down (in bed if you like – this is a great bedtime meditation). Take a few deep breaths from your belly.

2\.
Bring your awareness to your feet and observe any sensations. If you notice any discomfort, acknowledge it and gently breathe through it.

3\.
Visualise any tension leaving your body through your breath. Move on when you feel ready.

4\.
Continue upwards to your calves in the same way, then your knees and each area of your body, moving gradually upwards until you reach the top of your head.

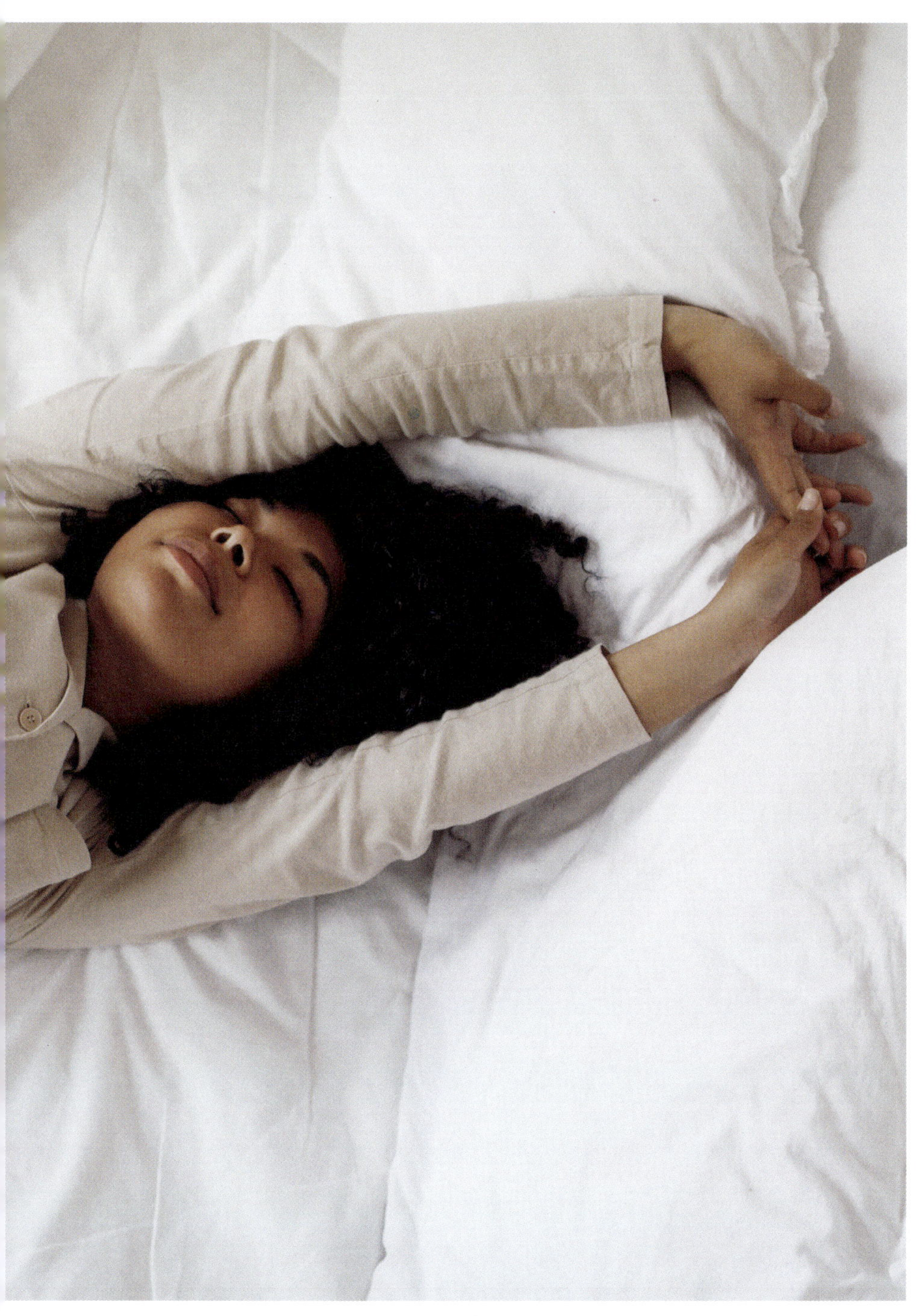

AFFIRMATION

I am grateful for the love and connection in my life.

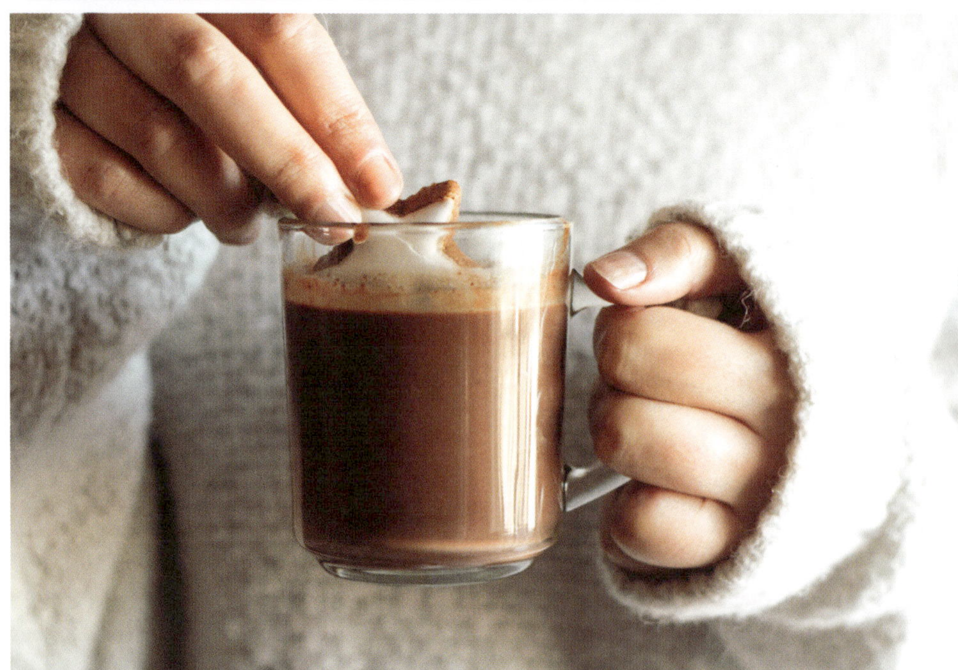

Luscious Hot Chocolate

Nothing accompanies a deep and meaningful conversation better than a mug of sweet hot chocolate. Make it for a friend and open your heart.

INGREDIENTS

4 cups whole milk

¼ cup unsweetened cocoa powder

¼ cup raw sugar

½ cup dark chocolate chips or chopped chocolate bar

¼ teaspoon pure vanilla extract

METHOD

Put milk, cocoa powder and sugar in a small saucepan. Heat over medium-low heat, whisking frequently, until warm but not boiling. Add chocolate chips and whisk constantly until the chocolate chips melt completely. Whisk in vanilla extract and serve immediately.

The Dog

"Man's best friend" earned his title through endless loyalty, complete devotion and unconditional love.

There is no love like a dog's love. Dogs ask no questions and make no judgements – they know simply that they want to be with you, whatever you're doing.

Dogs remind us to be pure of heart in our relationships. That doesn't mean letting people take advantage of our good nature, but viewing others with compassion and understanding. It means sticking by those we love in good times and in bad. It means giving friendship and affection and expecting nothing in return.

If you're feeling lonely and in need of companionship, get your hands on a dog and spend some quality playtime together. That trusting doggy energy will open your heart and get your love vibes flowing.

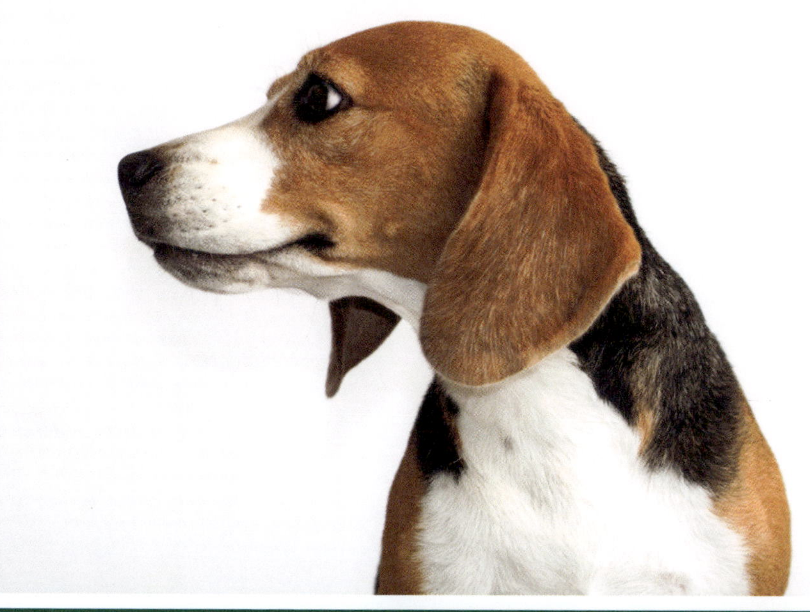

FAMOUS DOGS WE KNOW BY NAME

Lassie

Benji

Toto

Marley

Slink

Doug the Pug

Scooby-Doo

Lady and the Tramp

Santa's Little Helper

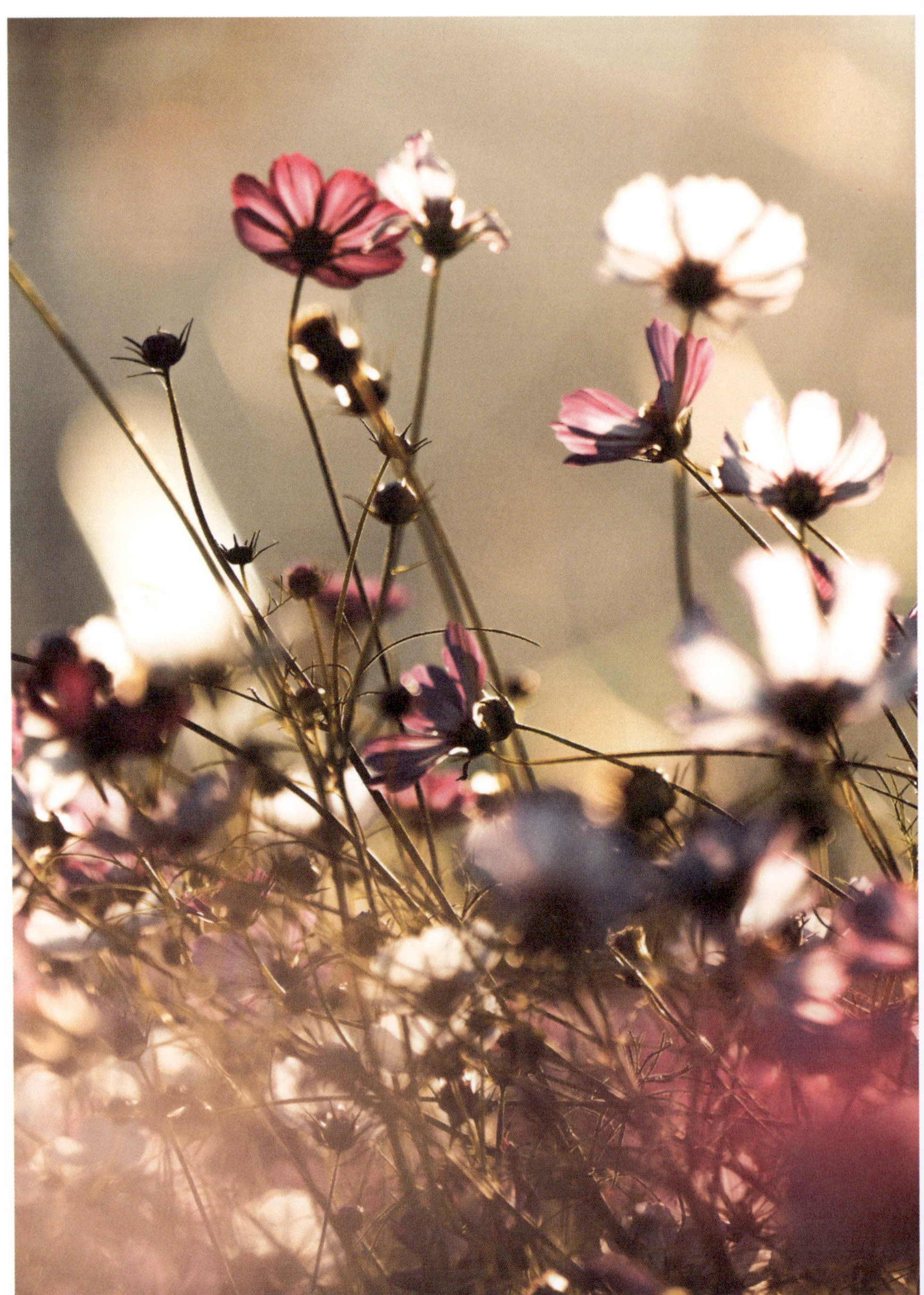

"WHEN YOU LIKE A FLOWER, YOU JUST PLUCK IT. BUT WHEN YOU LOVE A FLOWER, YOU WATER IT DAILY."

— ANONYMOUS

CHAPTER FIVE

Disconnect xx

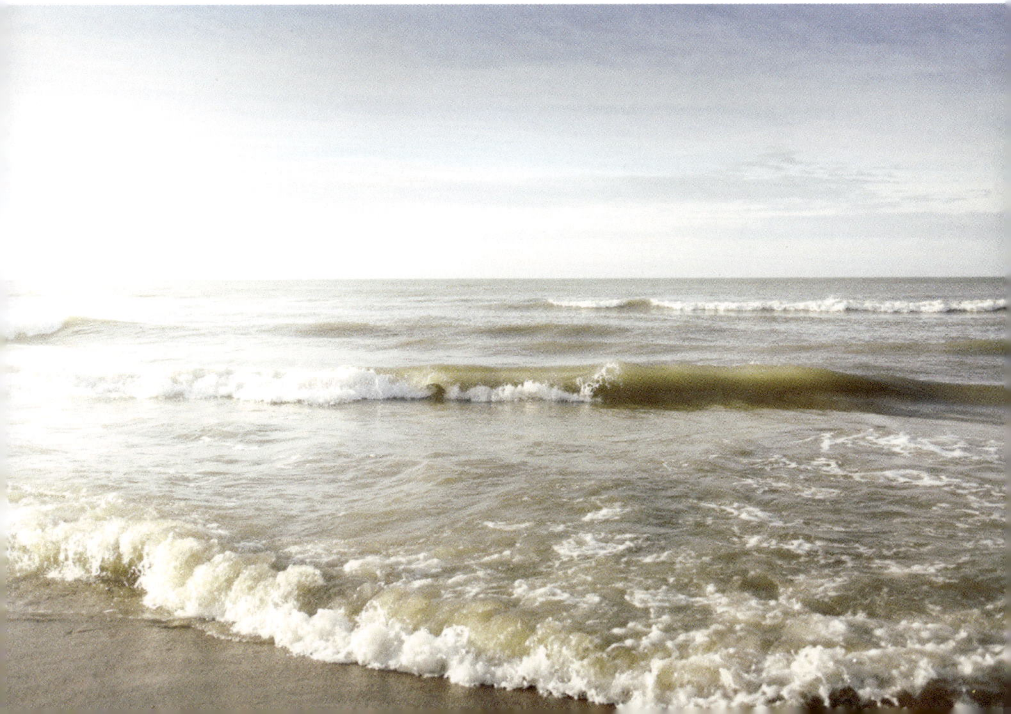

"Life is what happens when you put your phone away."

— ANONYMOUS

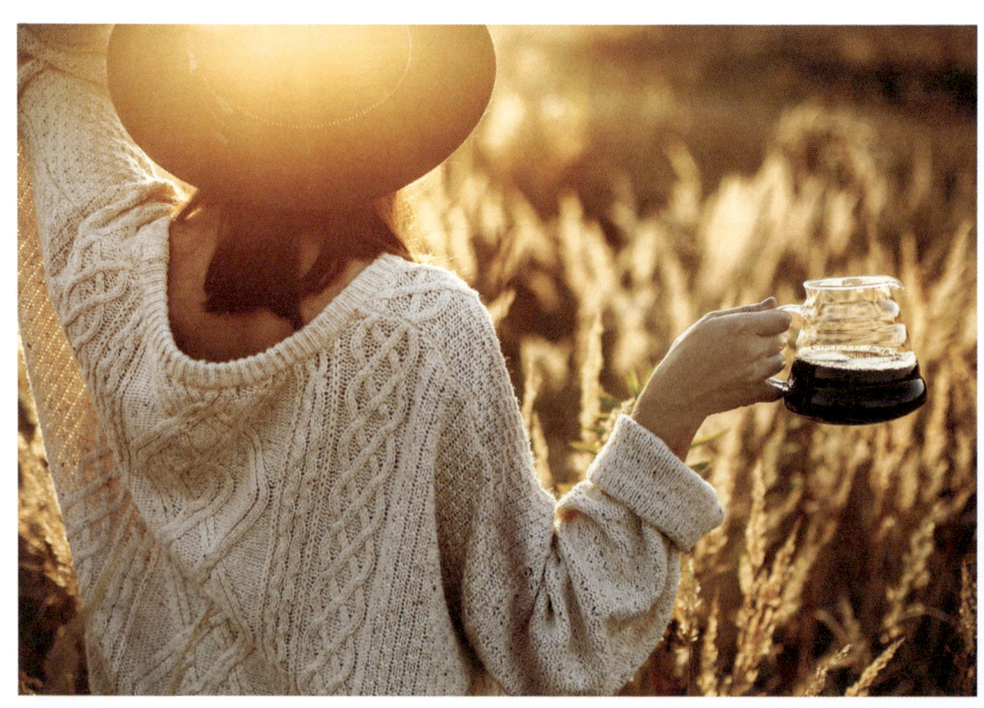

Get real

Isn't it ironic?

In many ways, we've never been more connected. Social media, messaging apps – it's easier than it's ever been to connect with people remotely, to follow distant events, to create virtual communities.

There are huge benefits to our online lives. It's when online becomes our lifeline that it becomes a problem. Virtual relationships can't replace good old IRL when it comes to human connection. Reading someone's eyes, nurturing human touch and the natural ebb and flow of a long conversation – these are things that it's hard to replicate on WhatsApp or TikTok. Make time for them.

Living online can also take you away from yourself. Remember – your most important connection is with *you*. Disconnecting from technology gives you time for self-reflection and real relaxation, helping you feel more present in your life, improving your sense of wellbeing and calling you to nurture your relationships.

It's all about balance. Be aware of yours, and make space for the real.

What disconnection means to me

Use this section to explore the meaning of disconnection for you. Create your own definition of it. Who or what comes to mind when you think about disconnection?

My definition of disconnection is ...

"Part of maintaining your well-being is taking the time to disconnect from the outside to go within."

— DEEPAK CHOPRA

It makes me think of ...

I experience it when ...

My virtual life

Can you make a guess at how many hours per week you spend in face-to-face connection versus online or apps? What are the good sides and bad sides? Would you like to change the balance? Think about how you can make some device-free time in your schedule and make a commitment to yourself here.

Each week I spend ...

The positives of virtual connection are ...

The negatives of virtual connection are …

I'd like to change the balance by …

Start small and build up. Maybe you'll decide to disconnect for an hour a day, and gradually work up to a whole day a week.

Spring clean your socials

Social media can give us the feeling of connection without any of the real human benefits. If your Insta gives you more FOMO than warm fuzzies, it's time for a clean out. Scroll through your feed slowly. Pause, feel. Note down here the emotions you feel as you view these images.

"The purpose of a camera is to capture memories, not replace them."

– ABHIJIT NASKAR

Are there negative emotions in here? Have you found accounts that make you feel jealous, dissatisfied, uncertain? Unfollow. Add ones that give you a lift, a smile, an idea.

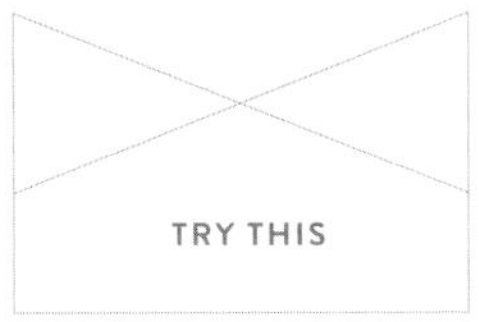

Stargaze

The experience of awe has been shown to increase generosity. It makes us see ourselves as part of something bigger, allowing us to connect more deeply with others. Gazing into the night sky connects us with the enormity of the Universe, helping us get things in perspective.

HOW TO DO IT

Set a date for the new moon, when there is no moonlight. Find somewhere quiet you can sit or lie. Breathe deeply, relax and look up, resting your gaze. Keep your eyes soft and open, not focused on any particular object. (Your eyes will take at least 20 minutes to fully adjust to the darkness.)

Notice any changes that you see in the sky. When thoughts, emotions and physical sensations bubble up, notice them and gently let them go.

Be in the moment

Mindfulness is pretty straightforward. It is the basic human ability to be fully present and aware of where we are and what we're doing. That's it.

It might seem trivial, but we're often in two places at once – performing a task while thinking about something completely different. Mindfulness shuts down our mind's chatter and allows us to just BE. We gain insight and awareness by observing our own thoughts, and we increase our attention to the wellbeing of others.

Mindfulness can be cultivated. And the beauty of it is you can do it anytime, anywhere. Take a moment to sit quietly and breathe, or practise while walking, or doing yoga or other sports. It starts with simply calling your attention to your body and being aware of exactly where you are and what your senses are telling you.

Think about how you can bring some mindful moments into your everyday.

"Life is a dance. Mindfulness is witnessing that dance."

– AMIT RAY

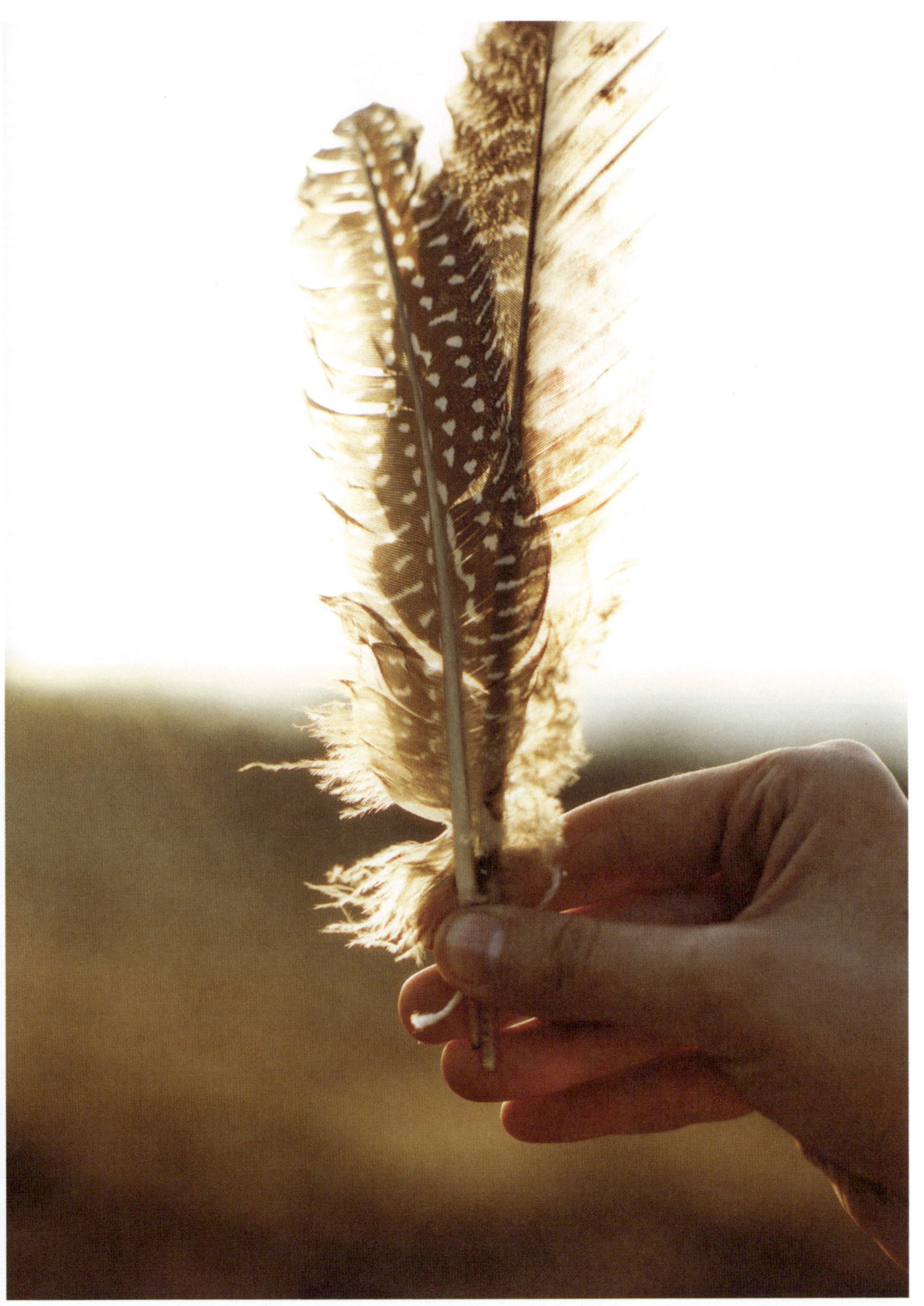

“Be where you are, not where you think you should be.”

—ANONYMOUS

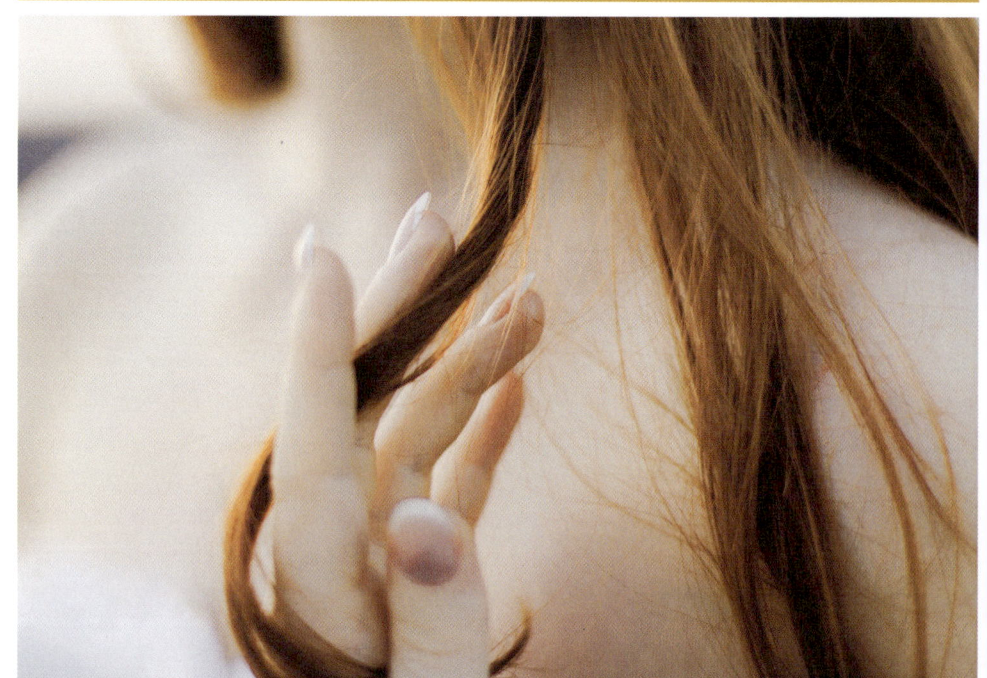

TOOLKIT

Disconnect

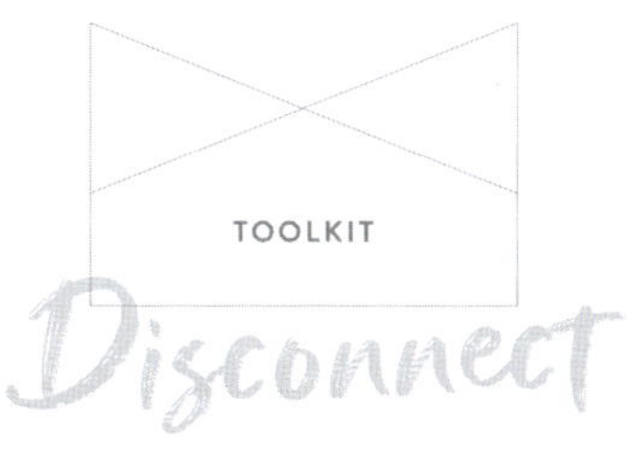

Sink into sleep with golden milk, find joy with a rainbow stone and chase a waterfall to find yourself where you really are.

AFFIRMATION

I am here. I am present. I am grounded.

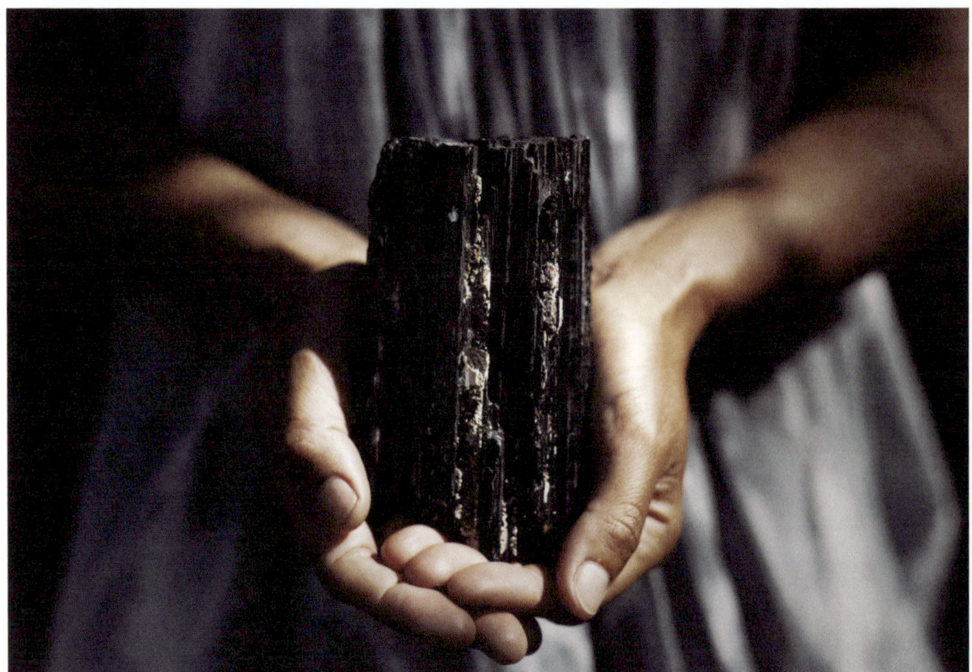

Tourmaline

FOR JOYFUL GENEROSITY

This grounding, rainbow-hued stone comes in glittering shades of black, green, violet and watermelon. Its colours ripple with imaginative play and generous sharing. It attracts inspiration, compassion and tolerance, and protects from negative energies.

HOW TO USE IT

A black tourmaline stone placed at an entrance or other strategic place will protect your home from dark energies and keep negative thought patterns under control. Place a pretty pink tourmaline sphere on your bedside table to radiate self-love and compassion through your dreams.

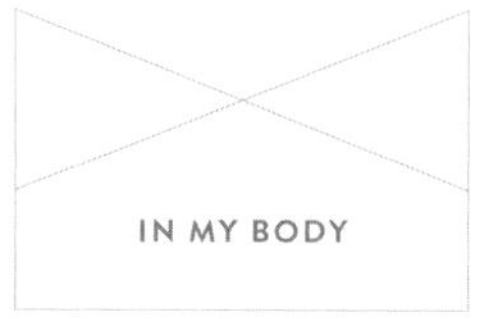

Meditation to Connect with the Moment

MINDFULNESS MEDITATION

A five-minute mindfulness check-in slows you down, stills the mind and calms the emotions.

1. Sit comfortably with your back straight and hands on your lap. Close your eyes.

2. Inhale and exhale deeply and regularly. Observe your breath flowing naturally in and out.

3. Be curious about the sensations you feel in your body. When your mind starts to wander, acknowledge it and redirect your attention back to your breath.

4. Stay here for five minutes.

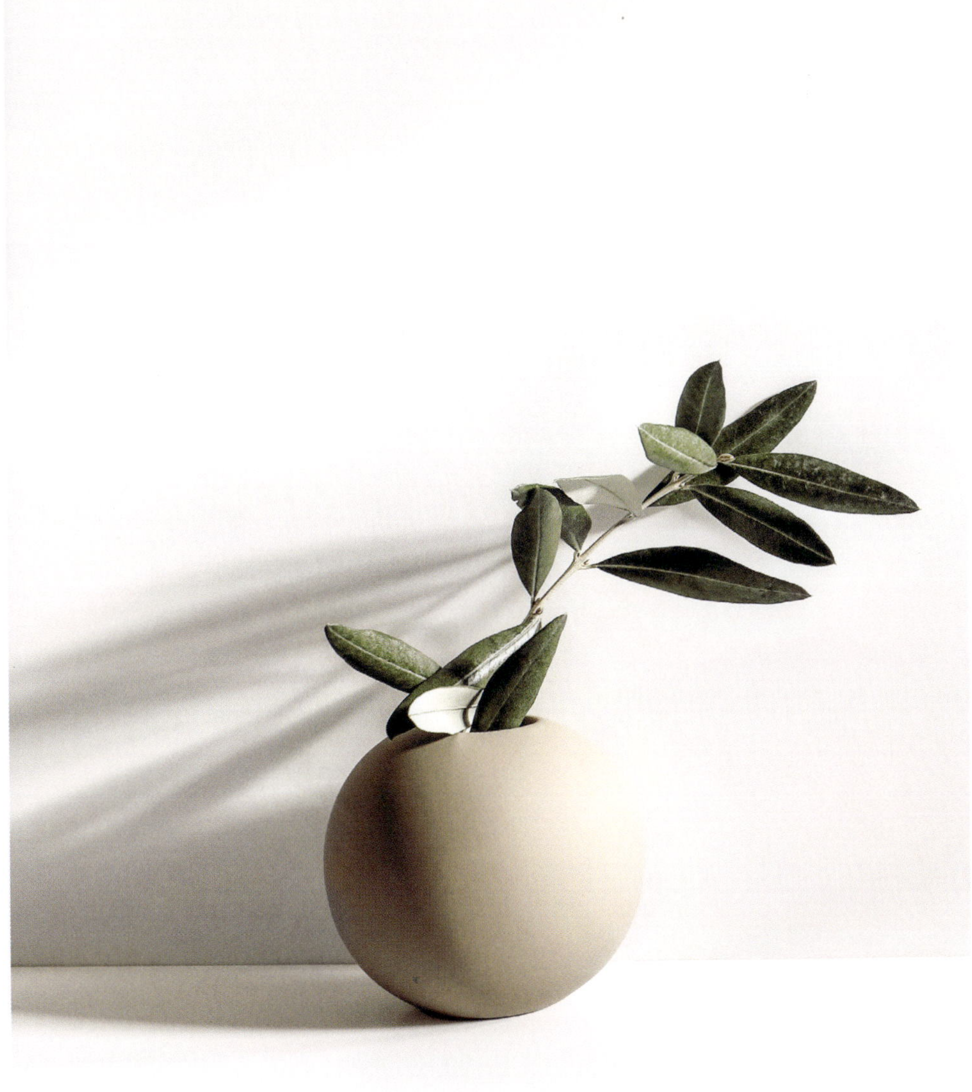

AFFIRMATION

In this moment, I have everything I need.

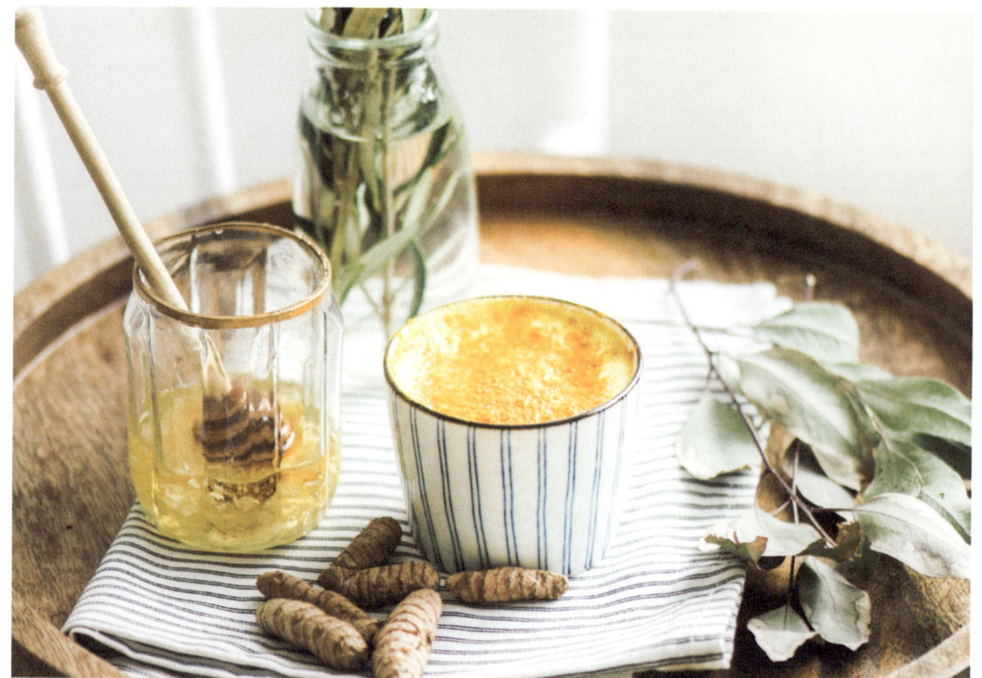

Golden Moon Milk

An ultra-soothing bedtime drink with roots in Ayurvedic traditions, moon milk aids sleeplessness, calms anxiety and supports the mind-body connection.

INGREDIENTS

1½ cups milk of your choice

½ teaspoon ground turmeric

¼ teaspoon ground ginger

¼ teaspoon ground cinnamon

pinch of ground nutmeg

pinch of ground cardamom

Honey (or other sweetener) to taste

METHOD

Bring spices and milk to near boiling in a small pot. Reduce the heat and simmer on a very low heat, uncovered, for five minutes.

Strain into a large mug. Add sweetener and whisk until smooth and fluffy. Dust with ground cinnamon.

Waterfalls

The rush of a cascading fall symbolises the flow of life and reminds us to accept with peace the rocky rapids – to go with the flow.

Think of the sound of a waterfall, both soothing and persistent. This white noise makes the perfect meditation soundtrack, pushing out thoughts of past and future so you can exist solely in the present moment.

Waterfalls are the kind of natural phenomenon that invoke a sense of awe, helping ground us and connect with the Universe. Naturally calming and emotionally soothing, they resonate with the symbolism of life's inevitable flow – there is nothing we can do to stop it, the best we can do is relax and go with it.

The waterfall reminds us to let go of expectation, exist in the moment and gratefully accept what life brings us – thirst-quenching mountain-fresh water.

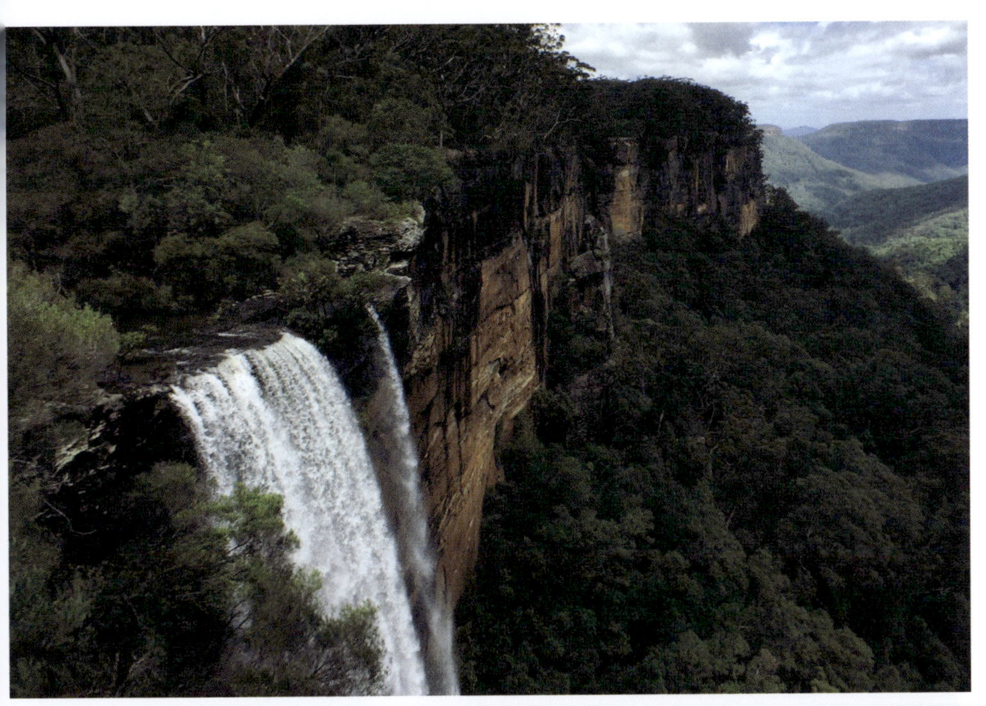

WATERFALL DREAM SYMBOLISM

Big challenges ahead

A fresh start

Releasing negative emotions

Regeneration and renewal

Hidden mysteries

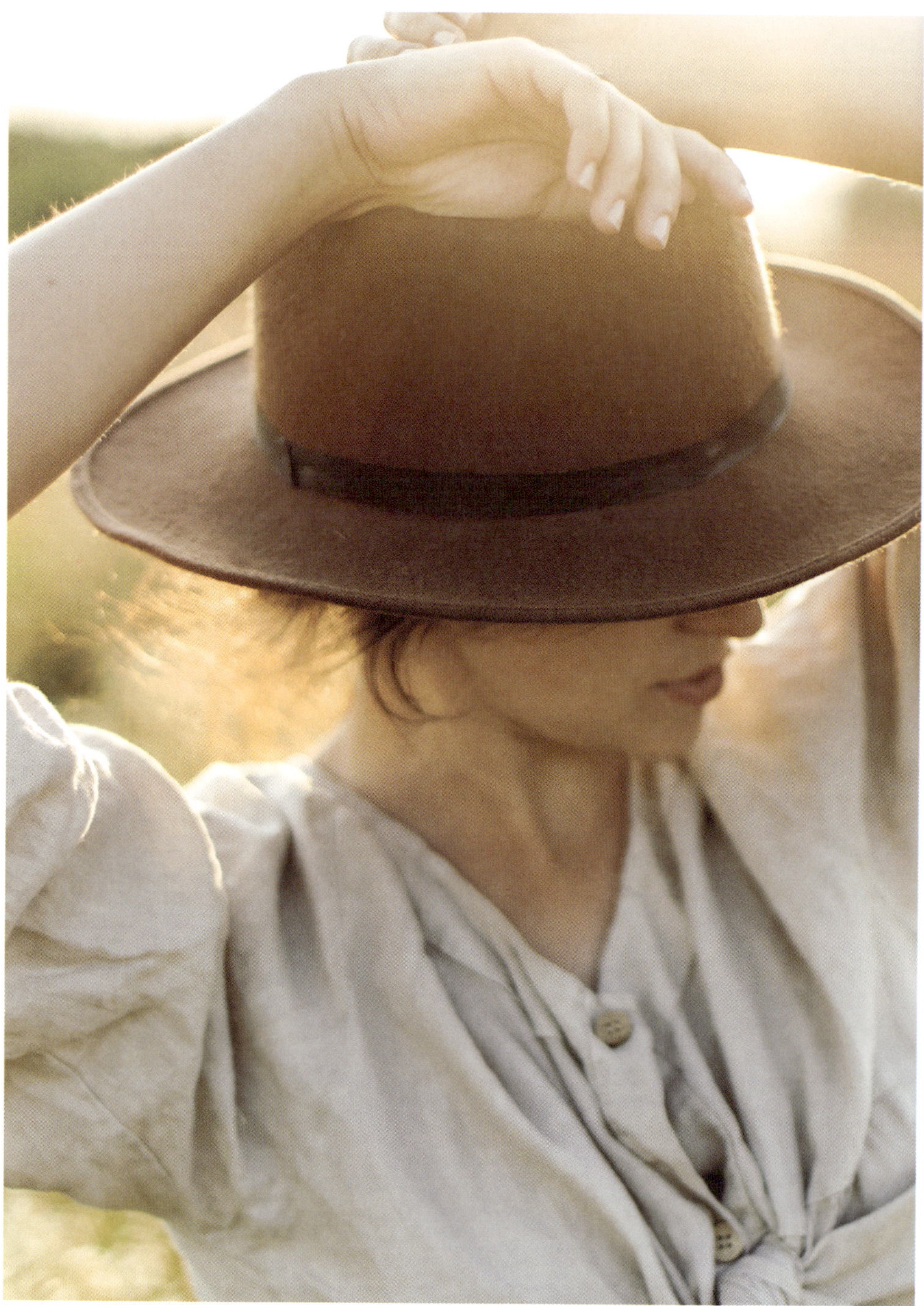

"WHEREVER YOU ARE, BE THERE TOTALLY."

— ECKHART TOLLE

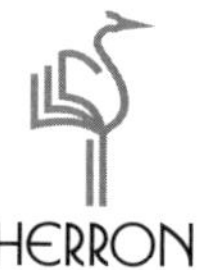

HERRON
First Published in 2023 by Herron Book Distributors Pty Ltd
14 Manton St
Morningside
QLD 4170
www.herronbooks.com

Captain Honey

Custom book production by Captain Honey Pty Ltd
12 Station Street
Bangalow
NSW 2479
www.captainhoney.com.au

Cataloguing-in-Publication. A catalogue record for this book is available from the National Library of Australia

ISBN 978-1-922944-22-1

Printed and bound in China

5 4 3 2 1 23 24 25 26 27

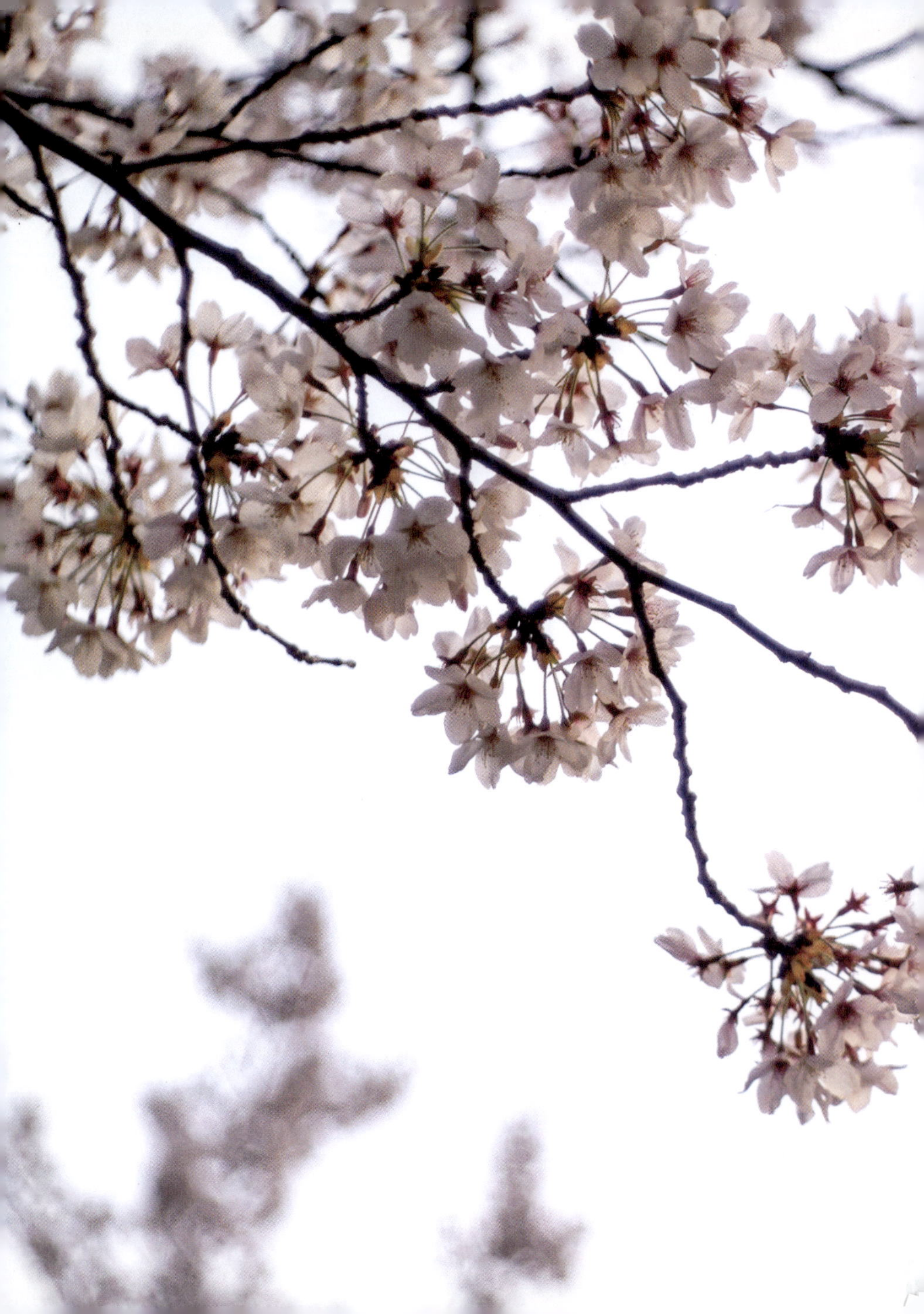